COLOUR GUIDE

Ob _ _ _ _ _ _

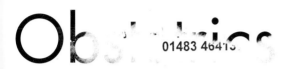

01483 4641

David James MA MD FRCOG DCH
Professor of Fetomaternal Medicine
Queen's Medical Centre
Nottingham, UK

Mary Pillai MD MRCP (UK) MRCOG DCH
Consultant Obstetrician and Gynaecologist
Cheltenham General Hospital
Cheltenham, UK

SECOND EDITION

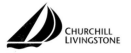

CHURCHILL LIVINGSTONE

EDINBURGH LONDON MADRID MELBOURNE NEW YORK
SAN FRANCISCO TOKYO 1997

CHURCHILL LIVINGSTONE
Medical Division of Pearson Professional Limited

Distributed in the United States of America by
Churchill Livingstone Inc., 650 Avenue of the
Americas, New York, N.Y. 10011, and by
associated companies, branches and
representatives throughout the world.

First published as Colour Aids—Obstetrics 1990
First Colour Guide edition 1994
Second Colour Guide edition 1997

ISBN 0 443 05773 7

British Library Cataloguing in Publication Data
A catalogue record for this book is available from
the British Library.

Library of Congress Cataloging in Publication Data
A catalog record for this book is available from
the Library of Congress.

Medical knowledge is constantly
changing. As new information
becomes available, changes in
treatment, procedures, equipment
and the use of drugs become
necessary. The authors and the
publishers have, as far as it is
possible, taken care to ensure
that the information given in this
text is accurate and up to date.
However, readers are strongly
advised to confirm that the
information, especially with
regard to drug usage, complies
with current legislation and
standards of practice.

For Churchill Livingstone
Publisher: Timothy Horne
Project editor: James Dale
Project controller: Kay Hunston
Design director: Erik Bigland

The
publisher's
policy is to use
**paper manufactured
from sustainable forests**

Produced by Longman Asia Limited, Hong Kong.
SWTC/01

Acknowledgements

We are grateful to the following for providing some of the illustrations for this book: Professor G.M. Stirrat, Dr B. Spiedel, Mr P. Savage, Dr P. Burton, Dr R. Slade, Dr D. Warnock, Dr A. Jeffcote, Dr N. Hunter, Dr C. Harman, Dr J. Haworth, Dr H. Andrews, Miss M. Freer, Dr S. Rosevear, Dr C. Kennedy, Dr J. Zuccollo and Dr J. Pardey. We are especially indebted to Mr N. Bowyer, of the Deaprtment of Medical Illustration, Southmead Hospital, Bristol, and Mr N. Bullimore, Department of Obstetrics, Queen's Medical Centre, Nottingham, for advice and practical help in the preparation of illustrations.

1997

D. J.
M. P.

Contents

Fertilization and implantation

Fertilization of the ovum by sperm occurs in the outer third of the fallopian tube. The division of the blastocyst reaches a 4-cell stage (Fig. 1) after 36–48 h. The blastocyst arrives in the uterus at 72–96 h (16 cells) and remains free in the uterine cavity for 4–5 days.

Implantation occurs 6–9 days after fertilization. Primitive chorionic villi develop at 13–15 days. The gestational sac is visible on ultrasound (US) (especially vaginal) by 4–5 weeks (Fig. 2).

Early diagnosis of pregnancy

For clinical features of pregnancy, see pages 5–8. Human chorionic gonadotrophin (hCG) is a glycoprotein hormone secreted by the trophoblastic cells of the placenta. It is present in the urine of pregnant women and is a useful marker for diagnosing pregnancy.

Detection of hCG, in practice, is undertaken using monoclonal antibodies. Such methods have improved the sensitivity so that a simple, quick kit test (Fig. 3) can now reliably detect as little as 50 mU/ml of hCG—the level found approximately 10 days after conception. *The expected date of delivery* (EDD) is 280 days after the first day of the last menstrual period (LMP) (Naegele's rule).

This method of calculating the EDD from the LMP assumes conception was 2 weeks after her LMP. Conception is likely to occur later with a long cycle (e.g. 35, 42 days), irregular periods or recent oral contraceptive use. Ultrasound (p. 29) may help clarify the EDD in such cases.

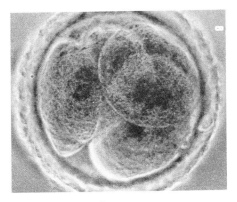

Fig. 1 Blastocyst: 4-cell stage.

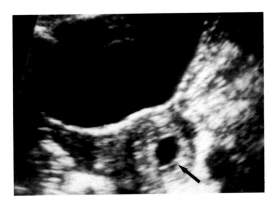

Fig. 2 US of gestational sac (5 weeks) (arrowed).

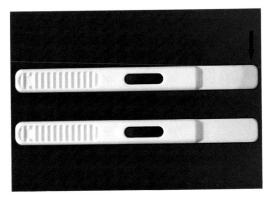

Fig. 3 Pregnancy test (blue is positive).

Fetal growth and development

The first 3 months of pregnancy (trimester) represent a period of rapid fetal growth and development.

Fetal growth

The yolk sac is seen by ultrasound (US) at 4–11 weeks. Fetal growth shows little variability in the first half of pregnancy when genetic control is dominant. Non-genetic factors give rise to greater variability in later pregnancy. Growth in the first half of pregnancy is recorded by US (Figs 4 & 5) using the crown–rump length (CRL) (8–14 weeks) and/or biparietal diameter (BPD) (from 12 weeks).

Menstrual age (weeks)	CRL (mm)	BPD (mm)	Fetal wt (g)
8 (Fig. 4)	15	—	—
10	33	—	—
12 (Fig. 5)	58	18	14
14 (Fig. 6)	80	26	36
16	—	35	97

Fetal development

Organ system formation is complete by 14 weeks (Fig. 6) (period of embryogenesis).

Organ system	Approximate gestational age of formation (weeks)
Limbs	6–10
Heart	5–10
Central nervous system	5–11
Eye	6–7
Ear	9–10

Pathology

hCG comprises α and β subunits. β hCG can be detected 9 days after conception. Approximate mean serum values are: 4 weeks, 1500 IU/l; 6 weeks, 20 000 IU/l; 8 weeks, 100 000 IU/l. The maximum level (11 weeks) is 120 000 IU/l, and 20 000 IU/l from 16 weeks. Fetal growth and development may be affected by factors including maternal diabetes (p. 55), infections (p. 15), drugs (p. 61) and genetic abnormalities (p. 25).

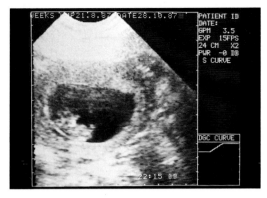

Fig. 4 US of 9-week fetus.

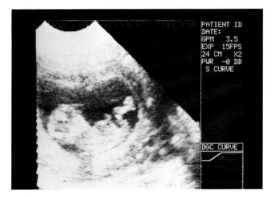

Fig. 5 US of 12-week fetus.

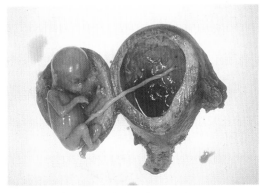

Fig. 6 14-week pregnancy hysterectomy specimen.

2 / Normal pregnancy and care

Aims of care

Pregnancy in most cases will be a normal event with low risk of harm to mother or baby. For a few, however, there is a greater risk of adverse outcome for mother and/or baby. The aims of antenatal care are:

- to provide appropriate surveillance to assess the degree of risk of harm to mother and/or baby
- for those at low risk with no significant problems in normal pregnancies, to provide advice, education and support
- for those at some risk of maternal/fetal harm, to provide additional care which will prevent, minimize or treat the problems.

Visits

Practices vary; minimum frequency is booking visits at 8–14 weeks followed by visits at 18–20, 24, 28, 32, 36, 38, 40 and 41 weeks.

History

At the first visit, the following data are recorded: maternal age, marital status, menstrual, medical and surgical, obstetric, family and social histories and details of any problems. Drug intake, alcohol and smoking habits are also documented. At subsequent visits any new problems are noted, together with maternal perception of fetal movements.

Symptoms

Amenorrhoea and tiredness are common early symptoms. Most organ systems may be affected in pregnancy—gastrointestinal (nausea, vomiting, oesophagitis, constipation, gum hypertrophy) (Fig. 7), urogenital (frequency), breasts (tingling, enlargement) (Fig. 8), skin (pigmentation) (Fig. 9), cardiorespiratory (palpitations, breathlessness).

Advice and support

The woman with a normal pregnancy is given advice and education during her pregnancy on diet and breastfeeding. She is strongly advised not to smoke or drink alcohol. ➡

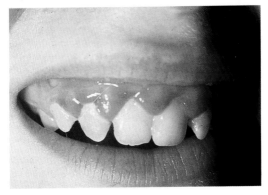

Fig. 7 Gum hypertrophy.

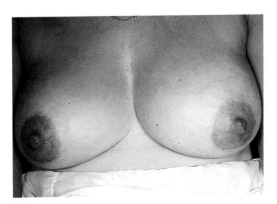

Fig. 8 Breast changes.

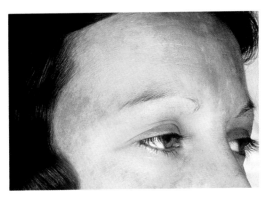

Fig. 9 Chloasma (facial pigmentation).

Examination	At the first visit a full general examination is undertaken. At all visits weight, blood pressure (see p. 51), uterine size, fetal number, lie and presentation are recorded. In later pregnancy the engagement of the fetal head is noted and the fetal heart is auscultated.
Signs	Early signs of pregnancy include changes in the breasts (enlargement, pigmentation, venous engorgement, and Montgomery's tubercles) (Fig. 8, p. 6) and genitalia (bluish colouration of vaginal skin and cervix, softening and enlargement of uterus). Other signs include: gum hypertrophy (Fig. 7, p. 6), chloasma (Fig. 9, p. 6), striae gravidarum (Fig. 10), linea nigra, umbilical pigmentation and eversion (Fig. 11), lymphadenopathy, thyroid enlargement (a soft systolic murmur may be physiological, oedema is found in 60% of normal pregnancies) and varicose veins (Fig. 12).
Investigations	At the first visit, urinalysis is undertaken (glucose, protein, ketones) and a midstream sample of urine (MSU) is sent for culture. Blood is taken for full blood count and film, ABO and rhesus grouping, antibody screening, rubella antibody status and serological test for syphilis. At 16 weeks screening tests may be performed for fetal neural tube defect by maternal serum alphafetoprotein (AFP) estimation and for Down syndrome (see p. 25). At subsequent visits, urinalysis is always undertaken and, for example, MSU at 30 weeks, full blood count at 26 and 34 weeks, rhesus antibodies in rhesus-negative mothers at 26 and 34 weeks.
Responsibility for care	There are two approaches to providing normal antenatal care: • all care is provided by an obstetrician • care is predominantly provided by a midwife and family doctor with referral to an obstetrician for problems.

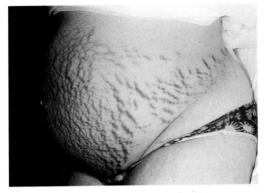

Fig. 10 Striae gravidarum.

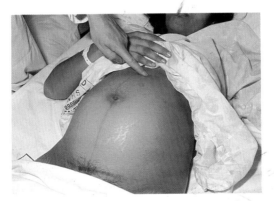

Fig. 11 Linea nigra and umbilical pigmentation and eversion.

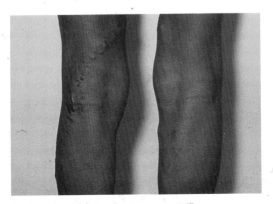

Fig. 12 Varicose veins.

Miscarriage/Spontaneous abortion

Definition	'Expulsion of the products of conception before the 24th week of pregnancy (20th week in USA) where the fetus shows no signs of life after delivery.' Most miscarriages occur in the first 12 weeks.
Incidence	15–20% of clinically detected pregnancies.
Terminology	*Threatened:* bleeding but pregnancy continues.
	Inevitable: bleeding, uterine contractions (pain), the cervix dilates and the products of conception are expelled (Fig. 13). It is *complete* when all the products have been expelled, and *incomplete* when not all the products of conception have been expelled (Fig. 14).
	Missed: the fetus dies but the products of conception are retained in the uterus (Fig. 15).
	Septic: caused by or associated with infection.
	Blighted ovum: an empty gestational sac with collapsed outline and no fetal node.
Aetiology	Most often none are apparent. However, if investigated, fetal abnormalities (especially chromosomal) are the most common causes. Others include infection, congenital uterine anomalies, fibroids, uterine adhesions, cervical incompetence.
Clinical features	Amenorrhoea, colicky pain/ache (40%), bleeding (98%), shock (5%), cervical dilatation and passage of products (15%), chance US finding (Figs 14 & 15).
Complications	Anaemia, shock, infection, disseminated intravascular coagulation, bereavement, grief.
Management	Complete, inevitable and some incomplete abortions may require no more than analgesia. Some incomplete and most missed abortions require uterine curettage. Blood transfusion may be required. Psychological support is important. ➡

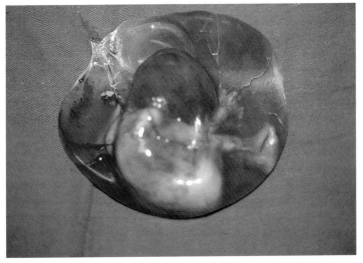

Fig. 13 Aborted abnormal fetus and placenta (14 weeks).

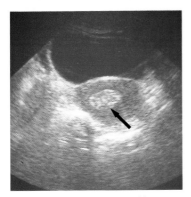

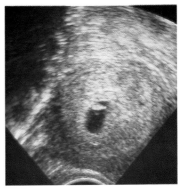

Fig. 14 Incomplete miscarriage with residual placental tissue in uterus (arrowed).

Fig. 15 Missed miscarriage: fetal size too small for gestation, irregular sac, no fetal heartbeat (vaginal ultrasound).

Defined as three or more consecutive spontaneous miscarriages. Causes include parental chromosomal rearrangements (e.g. balanced translocations), congenital uterine abnormalities, cervical incompetence, systemic lupus erythematosus, anticardiolipin antibodies.

Ectopic pregnancy

Implantation of a pregnancy in a site other than the normal uterodecidual area (1 in 100 live births). The most common site is the fallopian tube (Figs 16 & 17); others include the ovary (Fig. 18) and abdomen. More commonly found in women with intrauterine contraceptive device, previous ectopic pregnancy, history of pelvic infection (especially chlamydia) or tubal surgery.

Distension of the fallopian tube produces lower abdominal pain often unilateral. There may be some dark red vaginal bleeding due to decidual breakdown. Clinical features of pregnancy are not always found. On examination, the uterus may be soft and slightly enlarged, with positive cervical excitation and tenderness often with a mass to one side of the uterus. Tube rupture (approximately 10% of cases) will produce sudden pain followed by shock and collapse. Shoulder tip pain can be caused by subdiaphragmatic irritation by intraperitoneal blood.

Depends on clinical features, vaginal US findings and serum hCG levels. Options include:

Conservative: (asymptomatic, ectopic <2 cm, hCG <1000 IU/l): spontaneous abortion of ectopic confirmed by fall of repeated hCG values (some never adopt conservative approach if ectopic diagnosed).

Laparoscopy: (some clinical features, ectopic 2–6 cm, hCG 1000–15 000 IU/l): depends on size and site, blood loss and woman's fertility wishes. Options are:
- injection of ectopic with hyperosmolar glucose, prostaglandins or methotrexate; confirm success by monitoring hCG levels
- laparoscopic salpingostomy or salpingectomy.

➡

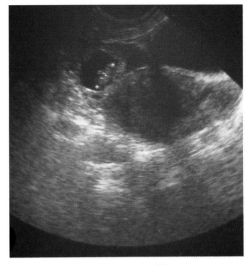

Fig. 16 Vaginal US showing ectopic with fetus above and left of an empty uterus.

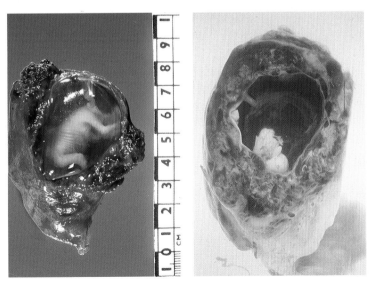

Fig. 17 Tubal ectopic pregnancy (opened).

Fig. 18 Ovarian ectopic pregnancy.

Laparotomy:	(shocked patient, ectopic >6 cm, hCG >15 000 IU/l): salpingectomy is preferred to salpingostomy. Blood transfusion necessary.
Sequelae	Increased incidence of subfertility (50%); further ectopic pregnancy in contralateral tube (10%).

Trophoblastic disease

Definition and incidence	'Neoplasia occurring in the placenta.' The incidence is 1 : 600 in the Far East but 1 : 2000 in the West. The villi become grossly hydropic with invasive properties and endocrine activity.
Types	The majority are benign (hydatidiform mole) although pseudomalignant, being capable of invading the myometrium and being carried in the blood. There are two types: complete (Fig. 19) and partial (Fig. 20). Very occasionally, a complete mole can become malignant (choriocarcinoma). A partial mole hardly ever becomes malignant but is always found in association with a triploid fetus.
Clinical features	Uterine bleeding, often after amenorrhoea, and exaggerated features of pregnancy are features of trophoblastic disease. In 50% of cases the uterus is larger than expected from the duration of amenorrhoea; in 25% it is smaller. There is a higher incidence of pre-eclampsia. Features of thyrotoxicosis are occasionally present. Villi may be visible through the cervix.
Diagnosis	Diagnosis is often made at curettage for presumed incomplete abortion. The levels of hCG are greatly elevated and ultrasound reveals a 'snow storm' picture of multiple cystic spaces within placenta. If a fetus coexists then the diagnosis is a partial mole (Fig. 21).
Investigations	Specimen for histology and karyotype; chest X-ray; serum hCG; thyroid, liver and renal function; full blood count; ABO and rhesus group.
Management	Initially the uterus is emptied by suction and curettage. Subsequent monitoring of urinary and/or serum hCG levels. Levels which fail to fall or subsequently rise again suggest incomplete evacuation, invasion, metastasis or malignant change. In such cases chemotherapy (the most common drug is methotrexate) is given. Hysterectomy is rarely indicated.

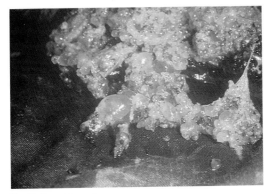

Fig. 19 Complete mole.

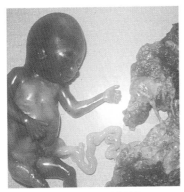

Fig. 20 Partial mole with triploid fetus.

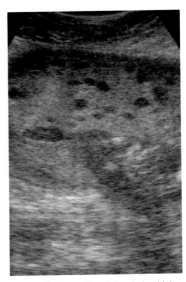

Fig. 21 US picture of partial mole (multiple echolucent areas in placenta and fetus).

Rubella

Mother

Clinical: Exposure 2–3 weeks earlier, 3-day maculopapular rash, lymphadenopathy, fever, malaise, conjunctivitis and cough.

Laboratory: Elevated haemagglutination antibody, specific rubella IgM antibody (falls after 3 months), virus from throat.

Prevention: Avoid pregnant women. Offer vaccination after pregnancy to susceptible mothers. Inadvertent vaccination in early pregnancy has not been associated with congenital disease.

Baby

Clinical: Permanent organ damage with maternal infection in 50% in first month, 22% in second month, 10% in third month and 1% after 4 months. Eye and heart defects, microcephaly, mental retardation, thrombocytopenic purpura (Fig. 22), hepatosplenomegaly, small-for-dates.

Management. Isolate (virus shed for 6–12 months), with careful assessment and follow-up.

Toxoplasmosis

Mother

Often asymptomatic, and there may be history of cat contact or raw meat ingestion. Diagnosis is by seroconversion, titre rise or placental histology (severe vasculitis and necrosis) (Fig. 23).

Baby

Clinical features include chorioretinitis, convulsions, hydrocephaly and intracranial calcification, thrombocytopenic purpura, hepatosplenomegaly, jaundice, fever, pneumonitis and small-for-dates.

If the baby dies, postmortem examination reveals that many organs can be affected by blood-borne spread: central nervous system (granulomatous lesions, pseudocysts, calcification—Fig. 24), eyes, lungs, heart, liver, spleen and kidneys.

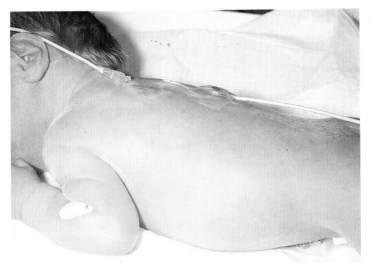

Fig. 22 Infant with congenital rubella showing fine petechial rash over back and buttocks.

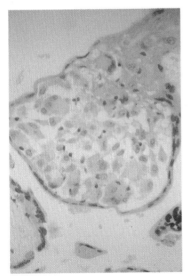

Fig. 23 Toxoplasmosis—placenta.

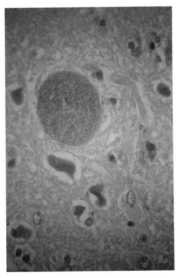

Fig. 24 Toxoplasmosis—fetal brain, microscopic appearance.

16

Cytomegalovirus

Mother

Almost always asymptomatic. If cytomegalovirus is suspected then isolation of the virus from cervix or urine is possible.

Baby

90% of cases are asymptomatic while severe fetal infection results in perinatal death. The remainder have thrombocytopenic purpura (Fig. 25), hepatosplenomegaly, chorioretinitis, microphthalmia, nephritis (Fig. 26), microcephaly, deafness, mental retardation, cerebral calcification and small-for-dates. Diagnosis is by virus isolation.

Histologically, CMV-infected cells frequently have cytoplasmic inclusions (virus particles surrounded by lysosomes) (Fig. 26).

Herpes simplex

Mother

Genital infection is sexually transmitted (see also p. 57). Painful vesicles are found on the cervix, vagina and external genitalia (Fig. 104, p. 58). Primary infection (multiple lesions and often lymphadenopathy) lasts for 1 week; recurrent infections (fewer, less painful lesions) last for 3–4 days. Diagnosis is clinical, cytological or by viral culture. Acyclovir has been safe and successful after the first trimester. Caesarean section is considered if delivery is anticipated within 2 weeks of active genital herpes or within 3 months of a primary attack.

Baby

Infection (from vaginal delivery with active herpes) can be disseminated (70%) (jaundice, purpura, respiratory distress, hepatosplenomegaly, encephalitis), localized (15%) (lesions on face) or central nervous system only (15%) (encephalitis).

Parvovirus

This virus can produce fetoplacental infection with fetal death due to hydrops (Figs 27 & 28).

Histologically, viral particles are seen as intranuclear inclusions in circulating erythroid cells (Fig. 28).

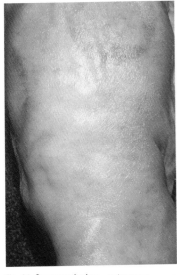

Fig. 25 Cytomegalovirus—cutaneous manifestations on trunk.

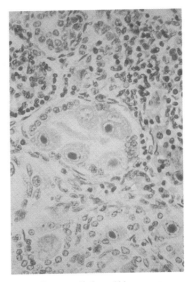

Fig. 26 Cytomegalovirus—kidney.

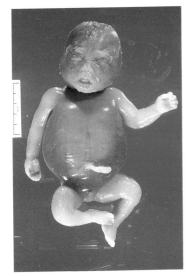

Fig. 27 Parvovirus—hydropic fetus.

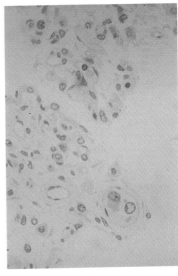

Fig. 28 Parvovirus—placenta.

Listeriosis

Mother

Caused by *Listeria monocytogenes*. The organism is commonly found in the gastrointestinal tract. Congenital infection only occurs with very heavy colonization. Listeriosis is usually asymptomatic, occasionally producing a 'flu'-like illness with abdominal pain. It very rarely presents as septicaemia.

Baby

Pregnancy may end in spontaneous abortion or fetal death. In survivors there are two types:
- *Early onset:* diffuse septicaemia with cutaneous (Fig. 29), pulmonary, hepatic and neurological involvement (mortality 90%). The babies are small-for-dates.
- *Late onset:* (possibly acquired after birth) meningitis with mental retardation and/or hydrocephalus (mortality 40%). Diagnosis is by isolation of the organism (Fig. 30); treatment is with ampicillin or erythromycin.

Syphilis

Mother

The risk of congenital syphilis varies with stage of maternal infection—50% with *primary* (chancre) and *secondary* (disseminated lymphadenopathy and rash); 40% with *latent* and 10% with *late* (gummas, neurological and cardiovascular). Diagnosis is by isolation of the organism (primary and secondary) and serological tests. Seropositive mothers are usually treated with penicillin irrespective of the risk to the fetus.

Baby

In severe congenital infection the placenta and fetus are hydropic and the fetus often stillborn (Fig. 31). Most are asymptomatic and may be seropositive or negative (recent infection). An uninfected newborn may be seropositive because of passive transfer. A few will manifest early congenital syphilis (Figs 31 & 32) (rash, hepatosplenomegaly, lymphadenopathy, oedema). Treatment is with penicillin.

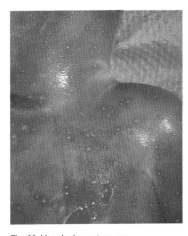

Fig. 29 Listeriosis—cutaneous manifestations.

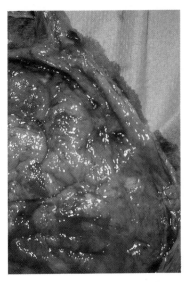

Fig. 30 Listeriosis—placenta.

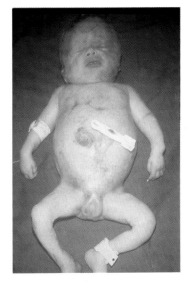

Fig. 31 Syphilis—fetus.

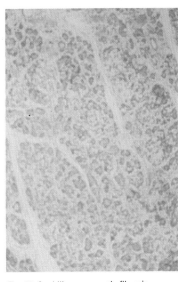

Fig. 32 Syphilis—pancreatic fibrosis.

5 / Prenatal diagnosis

General

Over the last 15 years dramatic advances have been made in prenatal diagnosis.

Obstetric procedures

These are performed under ultrasound control. Ultrasound is also the most important method in prenatal diagnosis (p. 29). The methods include chorion villus sampling (placental biopsy), amniocentesis, cordocentesis and fetal tissue biopsy. Such invasive procedures also allow fetal therapy to be undertaken, e.g. fetal blood transfusion for rhesus disease (p. 45) and in certain cases of urethral valves to insert a vesico-amniotic shunt.

Laboratory methods

These include chromosome analysis (karyotyping) (either directly or after fetal cell culture), DNA analysis, enzyme assay and measurement of haematological values.

Chorionic villus sampling (CVS)

Procedures

The method used can be by biopsy or aspiration using the transabdominal (Fig. 34) or the transcervical routes (Fig. 35). The transabdominal approach (using a technique similar to amniocentesis, see p. 23) is more commonly used than the transcervical route: it has a lower risk of miscarriage and can be used after the first trimester. After chorionic villi have been obtained (Fig. 36) they may be used for chromosome analysis, DNA analysis (e.g. cystic fibrosis, haemoglobinopathies, Duchenne muscular dystrophy) and enzymology (inborn errors of metabolism).

Risks

The risk is dependent on gestational age. The earlier in pregnancy, the higher the risk of miscarriage. Additional risks include membrane rupture, infection, rhesus sensitization and uterine trauma. CVS is rarely performed before 10 weeks because of the risk of limb defects.

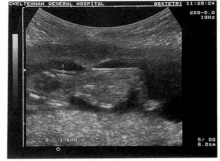

Fig. 33 Nuchal translucency (see p. 25).

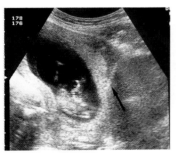

Fig. 34 CVS—ultrasound of transabdominal approach (needle arrowed).

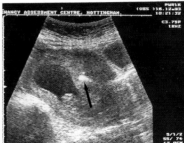

Fig. 35 CVS—transcervical biopsy under ultrasound guidance. Biopsy probe arrowed.

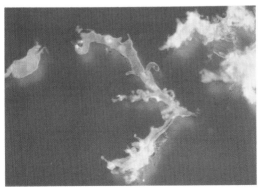

Fig. 36 CVS—low-power view of chorionic villi.

Amniocentesis

Procedure

Amniotic fluid is obtained by inserting a 20–22 gauge spinal needle into the amniotic cavity transabdominally under ultrasound guidance (Figs 37, 38 & 39). It is performed after the first trimester, usually at 16 weeks, though some are conducting the procedure earlier in the second trimester.

Indications

Chromosome analysis (for chromosomal abnormalities, fetal sexing in X-linked conditions), additional confirmation of neural tube defects (alphafetoprotein and acetylcholinesterase), inborn errors of metabolism (enzymes, metabolites using cells or supernatant), DNA analysis (where there is a gene probe for a specific condition) and later in pregnancy for assessment of rhesus disease (p. 45).

Risks

Maternal: delay for result (2–4 weeks with karyotype), infection, haematoma and psychological problems.

Fetal/neonatal: early—miscarriage (about 1%), trauma, haemorrhage, preterm rupture of membranes, labour and rhesus sensitization; late—respiratory distress and postural deformities.

Fetal blood sampling and other techniques

The aspiration of fetal blood, usually from the umbilical cord (Fig. 40) and after 18 weeks, is performed to diagnose inherited haemoglobin disorders, inborn errors of metabolism, karyotyping, fetal viral infection, rhesus disease, unexplained hydrops and fetal anaemia. Risks include miscarriage, trauma, blood loss, fetal death, preterm rupture of membranes and labour, and rhesus sensitization. Fetal skin and liver biopsy have been undertaken in the diagnosis of lethal conditions. Fetoscopy (direct visualization of the fetus) is now superseded by the above techniques.

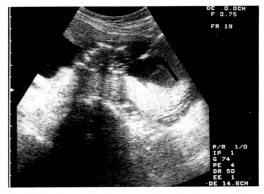

Fig. 37 Amniocentesis—ultrasound picture (needle arrowed).

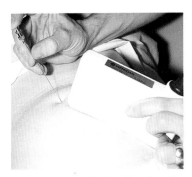

Fig. 38 Amniocentesis—insertion of needle under ultrasound guidance.

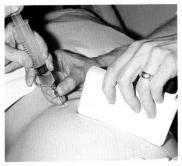

Fig. 39 Amniocentesis—aspiration of liquor.

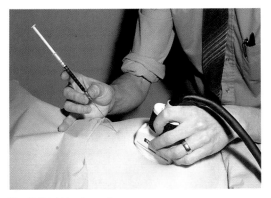

Fig. 40 Fetal blood sampling.

Down syndrome (trisomy 21)

Incidence

Occurs in 1 in 600 live births, and shows increasing incidence with older mothers (1 in 2000 at age 25, 1 in 365 at 35, 1 in 100 at 40). Overall recurrence risk is 1% (higher if there is a balanced translocation or if the mother is over 40 years of age).

Antenatal diagnosis

Diagnosis is by chorion villus sampling from 11 weeks onwards or amniocentesis early in second trimester. Discussed with mothers of 35 years or more, or with a positive screening test.
There is an increased risk of Down syndrome in women with low serum alphafetoprotein, low unconjugated serum oestriol and elevated serum human chorionic gonadotrophin. Screening is offered in many centres by measurement of these biochemical markers at about 16 weeks (65–80% detection rate; 5% false positive rate). Some centres offer screening by the detection of ultrasound markers (e.g. nuchal translucency at 10–13 weeks) (Fig. 33, p. 22).

Aetiology

Trisomy 21 in 94% of cases (Fig. 41), translocation in 3% and mosaicism in 3%.

Clinical features

Miscarriage/fetal death, small-for-dates, mongoloid facies, hypotonia, brachycephaly, single palmar creases, digit abnormalities, and often other congenital anomalies (e.g. heart) (Fig. 42). Mental retardation is common. Mean age of survival is 30–40 years.

Edward syndrome (trisomy 18/E)

Incidence

Occurs in 1 in 3000 live births; as with Down syndrome, increased risk with advancing maternal age. Recurrence risk is low.

Aetiology

Trisomy 18 (Fig. 43).

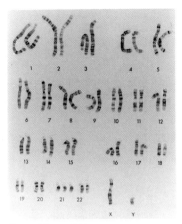

Fig. 41 Trisomy 21 karyotype.

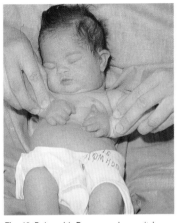

Fig. 42 Baby with Down syndrome (trisomy 21).

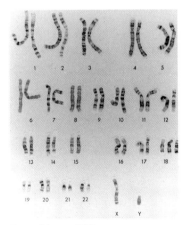

Fig. 43 Trisomy 18/E karyotype.

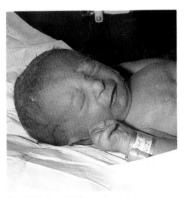

Fig. 44 Baby with Edward syndrome (trisomy 18/E).

| *Clinical features* | Miscarriage/fetal death, small-for-dates, severe mental retardation, hypoplastic lungs, flexion deformities, clenched fist with outer fingers overlapping the middle two, rocker-bottom feet, and craniofacial abnormalities (Fig. 44, p. 26). Other congenital abnormalities are common (cardiac, urogenital). The majority die within a few months; less than 10% survive more than 1 year. |

Patau syndrome (trisomy 13/D)

Incidence	Uncommon with a low recurrence risk. Higher risk in older women.
Aetiology	Trisomy 13 (Fig. 45).
Clinical features	Patau syndrome can present as miscarriage/fetal death, small-for-dates, midline defects of face, eyes and forebrain, holoprosencephaly, cleft lip and palate (Fig. 46). Severe mental retardation, deafness, rocker-bottom feet, polydactyly, congenital heart defects, and cryptorchidism. Less than 20% survive the first year of life.

Turner syndrome (45, XO)

Incidence	Occurs in 1 in 5000 live births; incidence is usually sporadic.
Aetiology	Single X chromosome (45, XO) (Fig. 47).
Clinical features	Turner syndrome can present as miscarriage or fetal death often with a cystic hygroma or hydrops (Fig. 48). Common features include small-for-dates, phenotypically female infants with transient lymphoedema of limbs, neck webbing, broad chest with widely spaced nipples, low hairline and short neck, and cubitus valgus. In approximately 10%, coarctation of aorta and mild mental retardation occurs.
Prognosis	Short stature, failure of secondary sexual development usually corrected with cyclical oestrogen from adolescence. Normally infertile. Cases diagnosed in infancy generally have normal intelligence and life expectancy.

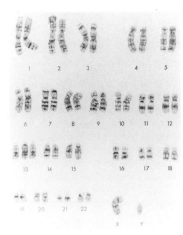

Fig. 45 Trisomy 13/D karyotype.

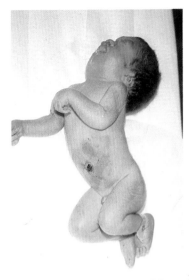

Fig. 46 Fetus with Patau syndrome (trisomy 13/D).

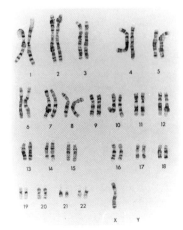

Fig. 47 45, XO karyotype.

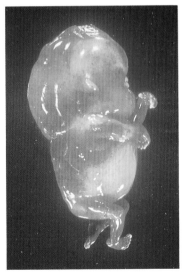

Fig. 48 Fetus with Turner syndrome (45, XO).

7 / Obstetric ultrasound

General

Approximately 90% of mothers in the UK have a routine scan in the first half of pregnancy.

Principles

A variety of obstetric real-time diagnostic ultrasound machines are employed (Fig. 49). They all work on similar basic principles with a probe (Fig. 50) applied to the maternal abdomen or into the vagina using a film of gel (to ensure good contact). There are two types of probe:

- a *linear* or *curvilinear probe* containing a series (about 40) of ultrasound transmitters and receivers
- a *sector probe* which has no more than three or four transmitters and receivers.

The identification of structures in the ultrasound beam occurs by the same principle as sonar or radar. Diagnostic imaging uses a $1\,\mu s$ pulse of ultrasound (usually $3.5\,mHz$) followed by a $1\,ms$ gap for detection of the returning sound wave. By sequencing the firing of the transmitters in rapid succession a real-time image is obtained.

Examples of the pictures obtained by these methods can be seen as follows: linear (Fig. 51), curvilinear (Fig. 73, p. 42), vaginal (Fig. 15, p. 10) and sector probe (Fig. 52). By incorporating a mechanism for detecting blood flow by Doppler ultrasound it is possible to get a real-time image with a colour picture of blood flow (Fig. 63, p. 36).

Applications

Determining fetal viability, diagnosing fetal abnormality, ectopic pregnancy, multiple pregnancy and trophoblastic disease. In the first half of pregnancy it is used to assess gestational age, and in the latter half of pregnancy for determining placental site and fetal presentation, documenting fetal growth and behaviour, and measuring liquor volume. It is a mandatory adjunct for invasive procedures such as amniocentesis.

Safety

The evidence supports the view that ultrasound is safe for mother, baby and operator.

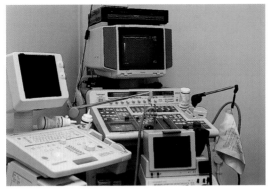

Fig. 49 Real-time ultrasound machines.

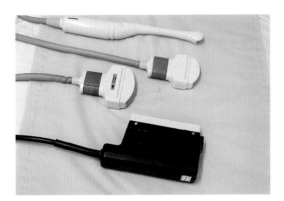

Fig. 50 Ultrasound probes.

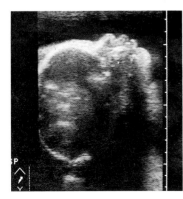

Fig. 51 Linear array scanner picture.

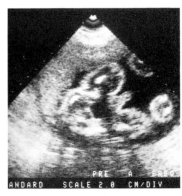

Fig. 52 Sector scanner picture.

Neural tube defects (NTD)

Types

Spina bifida (meningomyelocele, meningocele), anencephaly, encephalocele.

Incidence

Overall occurrence is 1 in 300 but displays geographical variation. In the UK the incidence in registered births has fallen by 90% over the past 2 decades. It has been estimated that at least 50% of this decline is due to antenatal screening programmes (see below) and selective termination of pregnancy.

Aetiology and prevention

Unknown but nutritional deficiency possible. Risk of recurrence (1 in 20) may be reduced if the mother takes folic acid from at least 2 months preconception and through the first trimester.

Antenatal diagnosis

Many areas offer mothers serum alphafetoprotein screening at 16–18 weeks. Elevated AFP ($>$2.5 multiples of the median) occurs in 80–90% of NTDs. Other causes of elevated AFP include fetal abdominal wall defects, multiple pregnancy, incorrect gestational age and bleeding in pregnancy. When the alphafetoprotein value is raised, a detailed scan is undertaken (Fig. 53). If then the diagnosis is still uncertain an amniocentesis is performed—a raised amniotic fluid alphafetoprotein and the presence of acetylcholinesterase would be diagnostic of NTD.

Spina bifida: a fluid-filled sac often containing neural tissue and an underlying defect of the spinal arch. 94% are lumbosacral. The degree of handicap varies and can include lower limb paralysis, urinary and faecal incontinence, limb deformities, hip dislocations, urinary infections, hydrocephalus (70%) (Fig. 54).

Encephalocele: herniation of the meninges and brain through the skull (usually occipital).

Anencephaly: absence of the forebrain and skull vault, facial distortion (Figs 55 & 56). Other abnormalities are common. Incompatible with life.

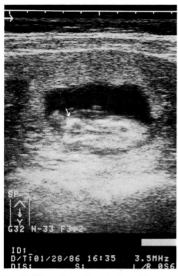

Fig. 53 US at 15 weeks; splaying of lower lumbar spine arrowed.

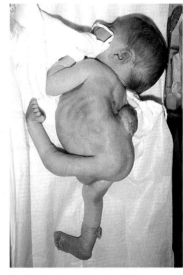

Fig. 54 Newborn with spina bifida.

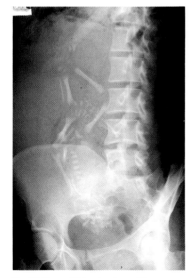

Fig. 55 X-ray of fetus in utero with anencephaly (no vault bones).

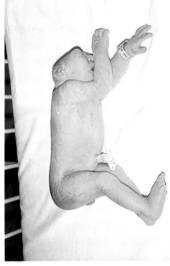

Fig. 56 Anencephalic baby.

Hydrocephalus

Definition

Excessive accumulation of intraventricular cerebrospinal fluid (Figs 57 & 58).

Aetiology

May be isolated, secondary to aqueduct stenosis or intraventricular haemorrhage. Most common associated abnormality is an NTD (and the Arnold–Chiari malformation).

Antenatal diagnosis

The alphafetoprotein is normal with a closed NTD. Diagnosis is made with ultrasound (Figs 59 & 60).

Prognosis

This varies. Babies with isolated defects may be born with accelerating rate of growth of the skull and a shunt may be required; even then the child may be irreversibly handicapped. If the hydrocephalus is not progressing at birth, the baby may be handicapped, although in many cases development is normal.

Intrauterine surgical procedures are of no benefit. If there is an underlying major abnormality (such as NTD), predicting the prognosis is relatively easier as it is generally poor.

Microcephaly

Definition and antenatal diagnosis

This requires ultrasonic demonstration of fetal head circumference below third centile for age and gestation which is disproportionately smaller than abdominal circumference and femur length.

Aetiology

Often unknown, but may be familial. Pathological causes include congenital viral infections and certain congenital abnormalities (e.g. Down syndrome). The prognosis depends on the cause.

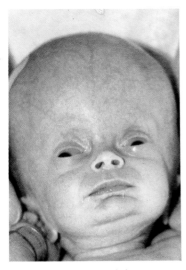

Fig. 57 Baby with hydrocephalus.

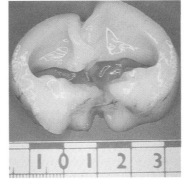

Fig. 58 Macroscopic appearance of brain section.

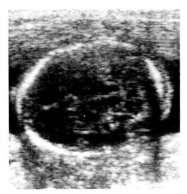

Fig. 59 Normal US appearance of fetal head.

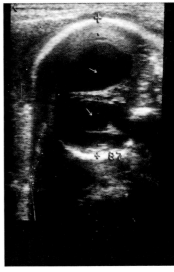

Fig. 60 US of fetal head showing dilated ventricles (arrowed).

Abdominal wall defects

Gastroschisis and exomphalos

Pathology

Uncommon conditions, with unknown aetiologies. Failure of rotation and re-entry of gut into abdominal cavity during fetal development.

Features

Associated with elevated maternal serum alphafetoprotein levels. Diagnosed by ultrasound.

Gastroschisis (Figs 61 & 62):   defect of the abdominal wall separate from the insertion of the umbilical cord. The abdominal viscera herniate and the peritoneal covering is lost (Figs 61 & 62). Usually an isolated defect.

Exomphalos (Figs 63 & 64):   herniation of the abdominal viscera through a defect at the umbilicus. Usually peritoneal covering is preserved and umbilical cord is inserted on to the sac. Other congenital abnormalities are common (cardiac, bowel and chromosomal). Karyotyping by placental biopsy or blood sampling (pp. 21–23) is advisable.

Management

Depends on associated anomalies. If not lethal, surgical closure is undertaken as soon as possible after birth. If a delay in operation occurs there is a danger of hypothermia and/or dehydration. This may be as a two-stage procedure, with the abdominal contents being enclosed in a temporary artificial sac initially. Mode of delivery does not influence the prognosis.

Prune belly syndrome

Incidence

Uncommon, with only sporadic occurrence.

Features

Deficient abdominal wall musculature, giving a rugose prune-belly appearance. Undescended testes and renal anomalies associated.

Management

Depends on the renal anomalies. If not lethal, abdominal wall is reconstructed in infancy.

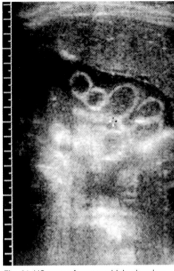

Fig. 61 US scan of gastroschisis showing loops of bowel floating in amniotic fluid.

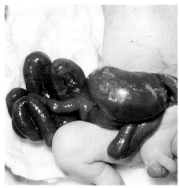

Fig. 62 Gastroschisis after birth.

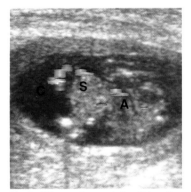

Fig. 63 US scan of exomphalos. Colour flow shows cord (C) inserted onto sac (S) on anterior surface of abdomen (A).

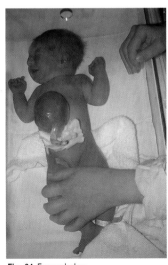

Fig. 64 Exomphalos.

Renal tract anomalies 1

Potter syndrome

Incidence Occurs in 1 in 3000 live births.

Aetiology The syndrome (Fig. 65) is produced by any condition resulting in oligohydramnios. Thus renal agenesis (the cause of the original description of Potter syndrome), dysplastic kidneys (Fig. 66), polycystic kidneys (Fig. 67) and urinary obstruction (p. 39) are urogenital causes. Chronic leakage of amniotic fluid can produce the same results.

Features Antenatally oligohydramnios, confirmed by ultrasound and also showing a compressed small-for-dates fetus. At birth, low-set ears, compression abnormalities with flexion contractures of limbs, and hypoplastic lungs. Possible renal failure with urogenital causes.

Course Death is normally due to respiratory failure (pulmonary hypoplasia) soon after birth.

Ectopia vesicae

Incidence Occurrences are very rare, although more common in males.

Features Wide separation of pubic symphysis with ventral herniation of the bladder, exposure of bladder mucosa. It can be diagnosed antenatally with ultrasound and is often associated with rectal prolapse, together with renal and genital anomalies (Fig. 68).

Management Surgical reconstruction is difficult. Incontinence is common.

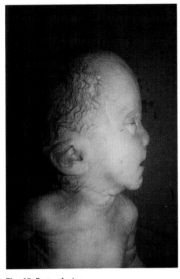

Fig. 65 Potter facies.

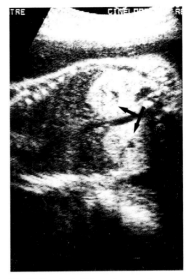

Fig. 66 Dysplastic kidneys (arrowed).

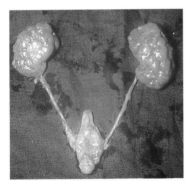

Fig. 67 Polycystic kidneys.

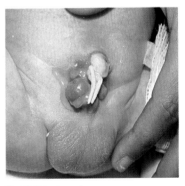

Fig. 68 Ectopia vesicae.

Renal tract anomalies 2

Urinary obstruction

Aetiology

Posterior urethral valves (males), congenital abnormalities of the urogenital system (such as a ureterocele) in females, pelvi-ureteric obstruction.

Features

Antenatally, oligohydramnios may be present, and severity depends on the site and extent of obstruction. On ultrasound, hydronephrosis may be seen (hydronephrosis may also be caused by reflux) (Figs 69 & 70). When the bladder outflow is obstructed, there is also a grossly distended bladder (Fig. 71) and sometimes urinary ascites.

Management

This depends on the cause, the degree of renal impairment and the degree of oligohydramnios. If the obstruction is mild, the renal function is normal in at least one kidney, and the liquor volume is normal, then the pregnancy is allowed to continue; investigate and plan definitive treatment in the neonatal period.

With severe oligohydramnios in mid trimester, the risk of Potter syndrome (see p. 37) is high.

In some cases assessment of renal function (by, for example, fetal urinary electrolyte examination on urine obtained by US guided needling) may be undertaken prior to the insertion of a vesico-amniotic shunt to try to preserve kidney function, restore liquor volume and prevent pulmonary hypoplasia (Fig. 72). In such cases, however, it would be wise to exclude chromosomal abnormality by placental biopsy (CVS) or fetal blood sampling (pp. 21–23) before undertaking the procedure. (Diagnostic difficulty may also arise in differentiating the oligohydramnios of renal origin from that due to severe early placental dysfunction.)

In many severe cases however, especially those presenting in the first half of pregnancy, renal function is irreparably damaged and the outlook is poor (Fig. 71).

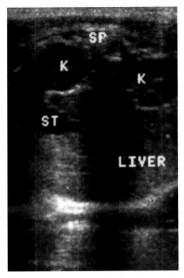

Fig. 69 US of transverse section of normal fetal abdomen (K = kidney; St = stomach; Sp = spine).

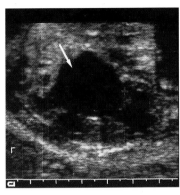

Fig. 70 US showing hydroureter (arrowed).

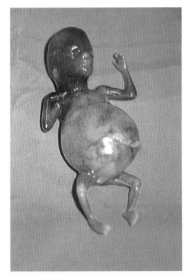

Fig. 71 Fetus with urethral valves and distended bladder.

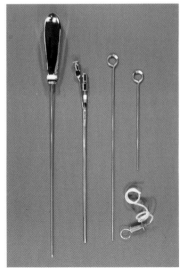

Fig. 72 Equipment for insertion of double pigtail vesico-amniotic drain.

Skeletal abnormalities

Osteogenesis imperfecta

Incidence

Uncommon. Varies in severity and inheritance. The severe congenital broad-boned type is autosomal recessive. Less severe forms may be autosomal dominant.

Features

Intrauterine diagnosis with ultrasound is possible. The long bones are deformed and shortened, and are poorly mineralized (as is the skull) with multiple fractures (Figs 73 & 74). Rib involvement may produce respiratory compromise (Fig. 75).

Prognosis

Varies from perinatal death to survival beyond infancy, but usually with marked handicap (deformities and deafness from otosclerosis).

Short-limbed dwarfism

Incidence

Many causes and forms. Achondroplasia is the most common (1 in 10 000 live births). Many are autosomal dominant (90% are fresh mutations). Severe forms (e.g. thanatophoric dwarfism—Fig. 76) are usually autosomal recessive.

Features

Short limbs, large head, prominent forehead. Severe forms have chest underdevelopment.

Prognosis

Milder forms: normal intelligence and life expectancy.

Severe forms: neonatal death.

Limb reduction deformities

Some are due to the amnion disruption sequence. There has been a recent suggestion that they may be a rare complication of CVS (p. 21). Thalidomide taken in the first trimester causes shortened limbs (phocomelia) with rudimentary hands/feet or absent limbs (amelia). The cause for most today is unknown, although can be found in association with other abnormalities. When bilateral it may be part of a syndrome involving haematological problems in the fetus associated with a high risk of malignancy.

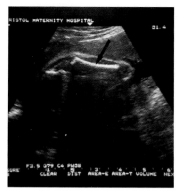

Fig. 73 US normal fetal femur (arrowed).

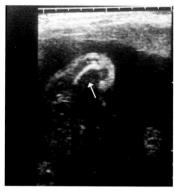

Fig. 74 US abnormal femur (shortening and angulation) (arrowed).

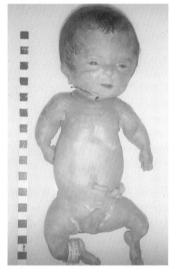

Fig. 75 Osteogenesis imperfecta.

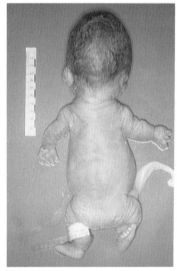

Fig. 76 Thanatophoric dwarfism.

Gastrointestinal anomalies

Diaphragmatic hernia

Incidence

1 in 1500 live births and caused by failure of fusion or muscularization of the anterior and posterior leaves of the diaphragm.

Features

Antenatally: diagnosed on US (abdominal contents in the chest and dextroposition of the heart) (Fig. 77). Karyotyping by placental biopsy (CVS) or fetal blood sampling (pp. 21–23) is advisable because of risk of associated chromosomal abnormalities.

After birth: cardiorespiratory compromise and scaphoid abdomen (Fig. 78). Clinical features and prognosis depend on size and degree of pulmonary hypoplasia (Fig. 79). Chromosomal or gut abnormalities may be found. Mortality is high (about 40%).

Tracheo-oesophageal fistula

Incidence

1 in 3000 live births. A developmental anomaly with oesophagus ending in blind upper pouch. Varying degrees of pathological communication with the trachea, bronchi or lower oesophagus.

Features

Hydramnios in 60% of cases. Diagnosis by absence of stomach bubble on US may be difficult because a fistula is present in 90% of cases and the stomach will not be empty. If suspected, the baby should not be fed until a gastric tube has been passed to test for gastric acid (absent with atresia).

Prognosis

Depends on the degree and associated anomalies. Surgical correction is usually successful.

Intestinal obstruction

Hydramnios is common. US may show a 'double bubble' with duodenal atresia (the first bubble is the stomach and the second the distended proximal duodenum) (Fig. 80) or 'triple bubble' with jejunal atresia, or 'multiple bubbles' with distended loops of bowel and peristalsis with more distal obstruction. Down syndrome may coexist with duodenal atresia. The more proximal the obstruction the greater the degree of hydramnios.

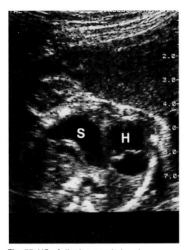

Fig. 77 US of diaphragmatic hernia—stomach (S) alongside heart (H).

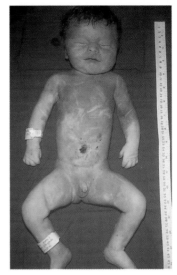

Fig. 78 Fetus with scaphoid abdomen.

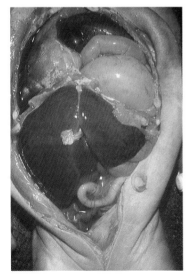

Fig. 79 Postmortem of diaphragmatic hernia—bowel in chest pushing heart to right.

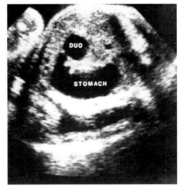

Fig. 80 US scan showing 'double bubble' of duodenal atresia.

During pregnancy

Aetiology

Five allelic pairs of genes determine rhesus groups (C, c, D, E, e). The normal rhesus blood group is determined by the D locus. Rhesus (Rh) disease occurs when a Rh-negative mother has Rh antibodies and a Rh-positive baby. The antibodies cross the placenta and cause fetal haemolysis (anaemia, jaundice (Fig. 81)) and, in the extreme, cardiac failure as hydrops fetalis (Fig. 82) and death. Rarely Kell or Duffy antibodies can produce a similar severe disease. Less severe disease can be produced by antibodies to the C or E loci, A or B antigens.

Sensitization

Occurs when Rh-positive cells enter the circulation of a Rh-negative woman (at delivery, abortion, placental bleeding, amniocentesis, CVS, external cephalic version or spontaneously).

Prevention

Prevention is by administration of anti-D immunoglobulin to Rh-negative mothers:
• at potential sensitization (see above)
• routinely at 28 and 34 weeks.

Detection

Unsensitized Rh-negative women are checked for antibodies during pregnancy.

Assessment

With antibodies, the severity of disease may be assessed by amniotic fluid optical density difference at 450 nm (Fig. 83) and, in some centres, cordocentesis for fetal haemoglobin (Fig. 40, p. 24). The timing of these invasive procedures is determined initially by the maternal antibody level, whether there is evidence of hydrops on ultrasound (see p. 48), and then on the results.

Intervention

With mild or moderate disease (e.g. A), less frequent testing and delivery at term. With more severe disease (e.g. B), more frequent testing; if the prediction approaches the action line, either delivery for neonatal treatment (p. 47) if not too premature, or intrauterine transfusion of blood if extremely premature or if hydropic with oedema, and ascites (Fig. 82; Figs 84, 85 & 86, p. 48).

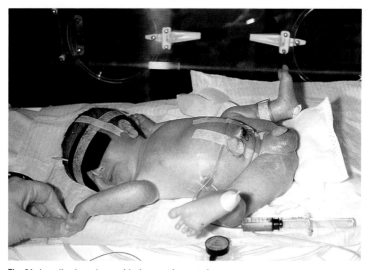

Fig. 81 Jaundiced newborn with rhesus; pigmented serum.

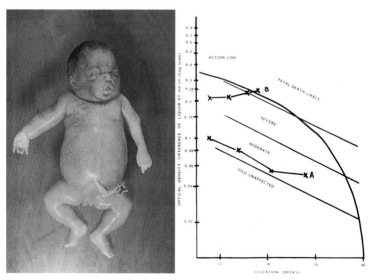

Fig. 82 Hydrops fetalis due to rhesus disease.

Fig. 83 Liley curve with examples of moderate (A) and severe (B) disease.

Rhesus disease

Testing at birth

Cord blood is taken for haemoglobin, Coombs' test and bilirubin levels.

Risks to the newborn

- *Haemolytic anaemia* (cardiac failure if severe).
- *Jaundice* (Fig. 83, p. 46) (kernicterus if unconjugated bilirubin levels are high).

Treatment

- *Severe anaemia*: exchange transfusion and possible anti-failure treatment (e.g. with diuretics).
- *Jaundice*: phototherapy in mild cases but exchange transfusion in severe cases.

Hydrops fetalis

Causes

- *Anaemia:* by haemolysis, though rarely before 20 weeks (Rh disease and incompatibility due to ABO, Kell and Duffy; red cell enzyme defects; homozygous α_1-thalassaemia) haemorrhage (twin–twin transfusion; fetomaternal haemorrhage) or marrow infiltration (Gaucher's disease); parovirus (B_{19}) disease.
- *Cardiac failure:* arrhythmias, cardiac anomalies, cardiac tumours and arteriovenous shunts (fetal or placental).
- *Hypoproteinaemia:* congenital nephrotic syndrome, hepatic enzyme defects.
- *Obstructed venous return:* neuroblastoma, cystic adenomatous malformation of lung, ovarian cysts, retroperitoneal fibrosis.

- *Miscellaneous:* congenital infection, chromosomal anomaly (e.g. Turner syndrome), chondrodystrophy, chylo/hydrothorax.
See Figures 84, 85, 86 & 87.

Management

The cause should be identified if possible, by ultrasound and investigating maternal and fetal blood. Even if a cause is found (80%), treatment may not be possible. Treatable causes include fetal anaemia, fetal cardiac arrhythmia and insertion of pleuroamniotic shunts (using the same technique for vesico-amniotic shunts, pp. 39–40). Overall survival is about 25%.

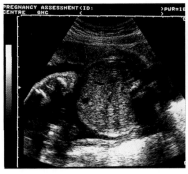
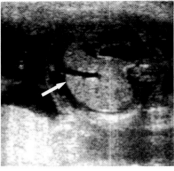

Fig. 84 US normal fetal abdomen (transverse). **Fig. 85** US fetal ascites (arrowed).

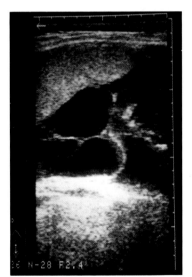
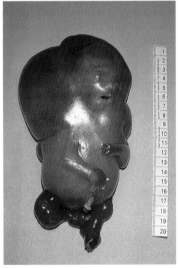

Fig. 86 US fetal head (compare with Fig. 59).

Fig. 87 Hydropic fetus.

Anaemia

Definition

The definition used varies but most definitions would include a haemoglobin less than 10–11 g/dl.

Aetiology

'Physiological' (due to haemodilution) (Fig. 88), iron deficiency (hypochromic, microcytic, low serum ferritin) (Fig. 89) and folate deficiency (hyperchromic macrocytic, low red-cell folate) (Fig. 90). B_{12} deficiency, infection, haemoglobinopathies and other causes are uncommon.

Prophylaxis

In many women, the daily iron requirement cannot be met by the diet. For such mothers supplementation with iron (100 mg elemental iron/day) and folic acid (300 μg/day) is recommended. The use of iron and folate supplements for all mothers is controversial.

Investigations

Once the diagnosis has been made, other investigations undertaken include red cell indices (mean corpuscular volume, mean corpuscular haemoglobin concentration), reticulocyte count, film, serum ferritin, red-cell folate and serum B_{12} concentrations, and electrophoresis if a haemoglobinopathy is suspected.

Treatment

Depends on the cause. Mild 'physiological' anaemia requires no treatment. Iron and/or folate deficiency can be treated with oral iron and folic acid together. The use of parenteral iron with associated anaphylactic risks (rashes, arthralgia, angioneurotic oedema) should only be given (preferably in hospital) when all oral preparations have been unsuccessful. Oral folic acid should be given with parenteral iron because of the stimulus to haemopoiesis. Blood transfusion in pregnancy should be a rare event (e.g. with symptomatic severe anaemia).

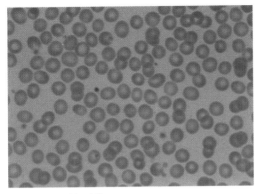

Fig. 88 Normal blood film.

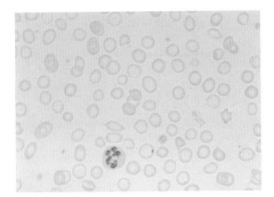

Fig. 89 Iron deficiency.

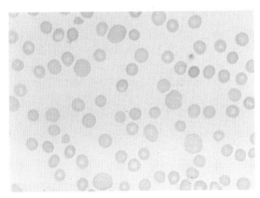

Fig. 90 Folate deficiency.

Hypertension (HT)—General

Blood pressure measurement
Semirecumbent/sitting relaxed mother, upper arm level with heart (Fig. 91) and conventional sphygmomanometer (larger cuff with obese women—Fig. 92). The diastolic blood pressure (BP) is the point of muffling of the pulse (Korotkoff phase IV). Different equipment (Fig. 93) may produce significant differences in recordings.

Definition
A sustained absolute systolic BP of ≥140 mmHg or a sustained rise of ≥30 mmHg over booking values or a sustained absolute diastolic BP of ≥90 or a sustained rise of ≥15 mmHg over booking values.

Classification
- Pregnancy induced HT alone ('PIH').
- Pregnancy induced HT with proteinuria ('pre-eclampsia').
- Pre-existing HT.
- Pre-existing HT with added pre-eclampsia.

Pre-eclampsia
Definition
A condition peculiar to pregnancy of unknown aetiology associated with multisystem endothelial damage and placental hypoperfusion. It is characterized by HT, proteinuria, renal impairment and fluid retention. Disseminated intravascular coagulation (DIC) may be found.

Types
- *Mild* (10% of pregnancies): after 20 weeks, BP <160/100, no proteinuria.
- *Severe* (2% of pregnancies): after 20 weeks, BP ≥160/100, proteinuria (≥0.5 g/l).

Associated factors
Primigravidity, previous severe pre-eclampsia, family history, pre-existing HT, migraine, diabetes, low socio-economic status, or any condition associated with a large placenta (multiple pregnancy, hydatidiform mole, hydrops).

Pre-existing HT
Causes
Essential HT, renal HT, adrenal HT, connective tissue disorders, coarctation, drugs (oral contraceptives, steroids).

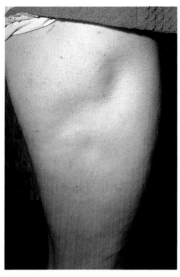

Fig. 97 Lipoatrophy of thigh associated with repeated insulin injections.

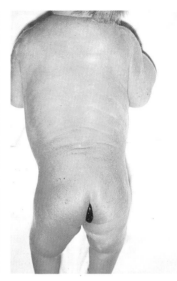

Fig. 98 Sacral agenesis.

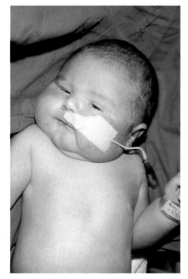

Fig. 99 Neonatal complications.

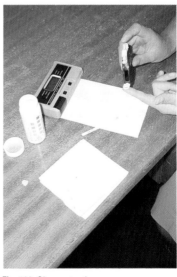

Fig. 100 Glucose testing.

Infections

Human immuno-deficiency virus (HIV)

Risk groups include women or partners who are drug abusers or from endemic areas of Africa, and women whose partners are bisexual or haemophiliacs.

Testing. Controversy exists over offering testing routinely for all women. Commonly those at risk are counselled and offered HIV antibody testing.

Risks to the fetus. Risk of transmission from HIV positive mother is about 30–40%; of these 30% will develop AIDS or AIDS-related conditions by 9 months. Risk of transmission may be reduced by giving AZT in the last trimester and by avoiding breast-feeding. It is still uncertain whether delivery by caesarean section is preferable.

Risks to the mother. Pregnancy does not appear to influence progression of HIV infection. HIV infection does not appear to adversely affect pregnancy outcome whilst the mother remains well.

Management. All women at risk, irrespective of testing or HIV status, should be managed as though positive. Vigilance and prompt treatment for infection. Extreme care in handling body products, especially blood, to avoid skin contact. Advise against breast-feeding in developed countries.

Candidiasis

Usually presents as pruritus vulvae, white discharge and erythema (Fig. 101). Treated with an antifungal agent (e.g. miconazole, clotrimazole).

Trichomoniasis

Trichomonas vaginalis produces pruritus and green frothy vaginal discharge. Oral metronidazole should be given to mother and male partner.

Gonorrhoea

Neisseria gonorrhoeae (Fig. 102) attacks columnar and transitional epithelium (e.g. urethra, endocervix and anorectal canal). May be asymptomatic but usually presents with a purulent discharge from urethra or cervix. The baby can become infected during delivery and develop conjunctivitis (Fig. 103), arthritis, meningitis or generalized septicaemia. Treatment is with penicillin. ➡

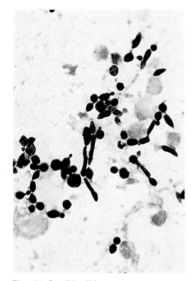

Fig. 101 *Candida albicans.*

Fig. 102 *Neisseria gonorrhoeae.*

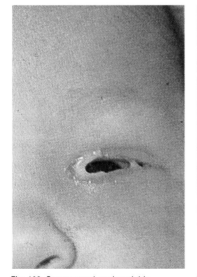

Fig. 103 Gonnococcal conjunctivitis.

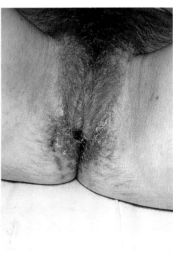

Fig. 104 Herpes simplex infection of genitalia.

Bacteriuria is significant when there are $>10^5$ organisms/ml of cultured urine (5% of pregnancies). Association with preterm delivery and anaemia. *E. coli* is the organism in 90% of cases. May present as:
- *lower infection* (asymptomatic or cystitis); outpatient treatment with oral antibiotics and liberal fluid intake
- *upper infection* (pyelonephritis); in-patient treatment with i.v. fluids and i.v. antibiotics.

Dermatological problems

The skin manifestations of systemic lupus erythematosus (SLE), dermatomyositis and systemic sclerosis can recur in pregnancy, requiring treatment with oral steroids. Risk of fetal growth retardation and death is more common with all three conditions.

Eczema and psoriasis can worsen or improve in pregnancy. Non-pregnancy treatments can be used for worsening disease.

Pruritus gravidarum is itching secondary to pregnancy related intrahepatic cholestasis (0.2% pregnancies). Recurrent in 40% of cases. Increased risk of prematurity and stillbirth. Diagnosis is by elevation of serum bile acids. Control can be achieved with urodesoxycholic acid (not yet licenced for pregnancy). Delivery is the cure.

Specific dermatoses of pregnancy include polymorphic eruption (Fig. 105) (0.75% incidence, erythematous oedematous papules); pruritic folliculitis (Fig. 106) (pruritic erythematous follicular papules); prurigo (Fig. 107) (0.3% incidence, itchy excoriated papules); pemphigoid ('herpes') gestationis (Fig. 108) (1:50000 incidence, recurrent condition associated with autoimmune conditions, pruritic urticarial papules, vesicles and bullae). The distribution is especially over abdomen and thighs. Treatment with oral antihistamines and topical 1% hydrocortisone is usually effective.

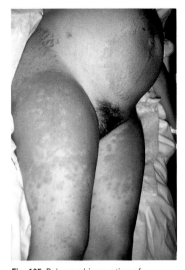

Fig. 105 Polymorphic eruption of pregnancy.

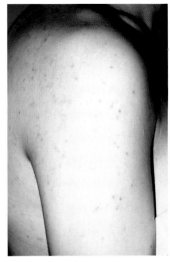

Fig. 106 Pruritic folliculitis of pregnancy.

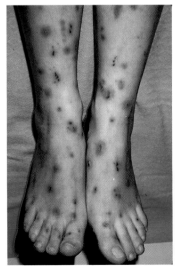

Fig. 107 Prurigo of pregnancy.

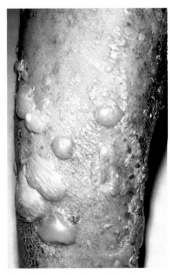

Fig. 108 Pemphigoid gestationis.

Prescribed drugs

Most drugs both cross the placenta and are excreted in breast milk. In the first trimester the theoretical risk of congenital malformations is only proven for a few drugs. Fetal growth and development can be affected later (e.g. tetracycline-staining of fetal teeth—Fig. 109; antithyroid agents and fetal goitre—Fig. 110). Some drugs given close to term or in labour can affect the newborn (e.g. narcotic analgesia and neonatal depression). Drugs should only be prescribed where there are clear indications. Drug therapy in the first trimester should be avoided if at all possible.

Smoking

Maternal smoking (20 cigarettes/day) reduces the mean birthweight by 200–300 g. It is synergistic with the effect of alcohol. It is prevented by stopping smoking in the second half of pregnancy. Maternal smoking during pregnancy also increases the risk of sudden infant death.

Alcohol

Excessive chronic alcohol consumption ($\geq$80 g/day), (10 g is a 0.5 pint, a 'short', a glass of wine or a sherry) may cause the fetal alcohol syndrome (Fig. 111): mental retardation, growth retardation, characteristic facies with short palpebral fissures, hypoplastic nasal philtrum and micrognathia. Fetal growth retardation alone is a more consistent finding with an alcohol consumption of $\geq$40 g/day.

Drug abuse

Complications more common in women who abuse drugs during pregnancy include anaemia; premature membrane rupture; antepartum haemorrhage; multiple pregnancy; preterm delivery; fetal growth retardation; birth asphyxia and perinatal death. They are also at risk of hepatitis B and HIV infection. Neonatal withdrawal symptoms may occur, the timing depending on the drug and its half-life.

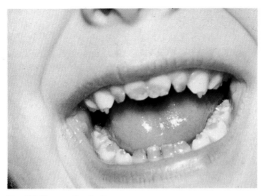

Fig. 109 Tetracycline teeth.

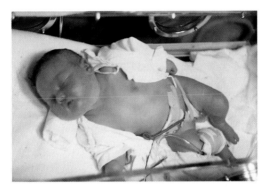

Fig. 110 Goitre due to maternal antithyroid treatment.

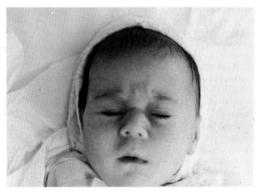

Fig. 111 Fetal alcohol syndrome.

Intrauterine growth retardation (IUGR)—Background

Incidence

About 10% of all live-born babies and 30% of those less than 2.5 kg suffer from intrauterine growth retardation. They have greater perinatal mortality and morbidity and later handicap.

Definition

'When a baby fails to achieve his or her genetic growth potential.' In practice, however, the diagnosis is not always easy as there are ethnic and geographical variations. The best definition probably is where a baby's growth velocity or trajectory on ultrasound falls below that expected for the normal population. It is important to note that fetal size does not have to fall outside the normal range for this pathological growth to occur.

Normal growth

Maximum velocity of linear growth occurs at 20 weeks, and of body weight at 34 weeks. At the end of pregnancy physical constraints probably slow fetal growth. Control is influenced by genetic and hormonal factors and nutrient supply.

Causes

Intrinsic: malformations including chromosomal (5–10%) and viral infections (2%).

Extrinsic: uteroplacental vascular insufficiency (e.g. pre-eclampsia), cyanotic heart disease, maternal malnutrition if severe (e.g. in famines), smoking, alcohol and idiopathic causes (30%).

Risk factors

Short stature, previous small baby, low weight (<45 kg), poor weight gain, multiple pregnancy, smoking, alcohol, raised alphafetoprotein, and other conditions (see *Causes*, above).

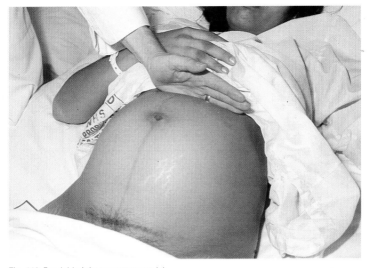

Fig. 112 Fundal height measurement (a).

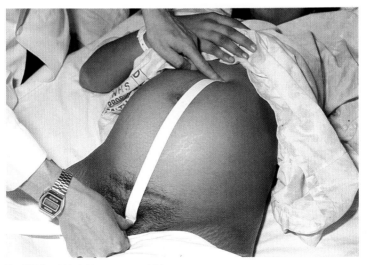

Fig. 113 Fundal height measurement (b).

Intrauterine growth retardation—Diagnosis and management

Diagnosis

This depends on a high degree of clinical suspicion based on risk factors. Nevertheless, 30–50% of IUGR fetuses remain undetected by clinical examination. Serial recording of symphysis–fundal height is claimed to be useful but this is not agreed by all (Figs 112 & 113, p. 64). Multiple pregnancy, polyhydramnios, transverse lie and maternal obesity reduce its accuracy. Assays of hormones (e.g. oestriol or placental lactogen) are no longer used widely. Ultrasound is the best method using the head and abdominal circumferences (see Fig. 59, p. 34; Fig. 84, p. 48 and Fig. 215, p. 124 for correct views for measuring circumferences). Two patterns of IUGR are recognized:

- *symmetrical/early:* usually due to intrinsic problems (e.g. congenital abnormality, viral infection). On ultrasound, head *and* abdominal measurements fall away from expected growth trajectories (Fig. 114).
- *asymmetrical/late:* usually due to extrinsic problems (e.g. pre-eclampsia, multiple pregnancy). On ultrasound, abdominal measurements fall away from expected growth trajectories *but* head circumference growth is initially normal (Fig. 115).

Management

The IUGR fetus should be scanned for congenital abnormality (p. 29). Cordocentesis (p. 23) for karyotyping, viral serology and (controversially) blood gases may be a necessary adjunct with severe cases. If normal then serial monitoring of fetal health is mandatory (pp. 67–69). The timing of elective delivery is determined by gestation and fetal health assessment. Doppler analysis of umbilical artery blood flow may be used to differentiate the normally grown small fetus from one with pathological growth due to uteroplacental disease (see p. 71).

Neonatal complications

Apart from major abnormalities, perinatal asphyxia, meconium aspiration, pulmonary haemorrhage, hypothermia, hypoglycaemia and polycythaemia (Fig. 116).

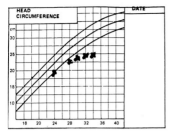

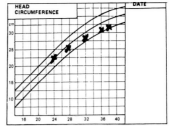

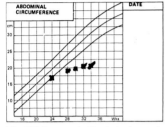

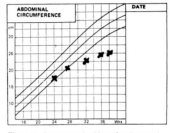

Fig. 114 Symmetrical/early fetal growth retardation.

Fig. 115 Asymmetrical/late fetal growth retardation.

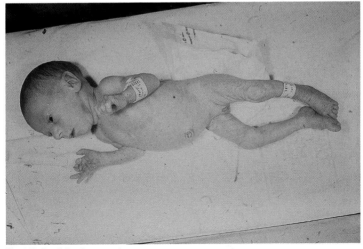

Fig. 116 Small-for-dates newborn.

Overview

Routine screening

Clinical assessment of fetal growth (Figs 112 & 113, p. 64) and noting maternal perception of fetal movements/activity. The fetal heart is also recorded routinely either by auscultation with a Pinard stethoscope (Fig. 117) or a fetal heart detector, using Doppler ultrasound (Fig. 118). The recording of the fetal heart in this way is a limited assessment of fetal welfare, being confined to answering the question of whether the fetal heart is present, and of normal rate at a given moment.

Biochemical and biophysical investigations

These methods are applicable to the fetus considered at risk either by using the above methods, because of a problem in a previous pregnancy (e.g. stillbirth), or because of ultrasonically diagnosed IUGR (pp. 63–65).

Biochemical assessment: is no longer widely used because there is a delay between sampling and obtaining a result. However, such tests might have a place in the future in screening. For example, a raised alphafetoprotein at 16 weeks without fetal abnormality is associated with an increased risk of IUGR, pre-eclampsia or preterm birth.

Biophysical methods: more popular. The underlying principle is that the fetus exposed to a chronic insult (especially hypoxia) will have a depressed central nervous system (reduced heart rate variability, movements, tone and breathing movements and, if severe, depressed renal function (oligohydramnios). The tests are the daily kick chart, non-stress fetal heart rate (FHR) recording (Fig. 119) and the biophysical profile (p. 69).

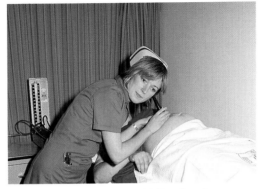

Fig. 117 Fetal heart auscultation with Pinard's stethoscope.

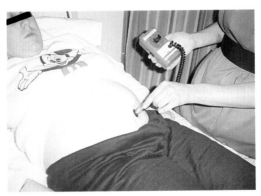

Fig. 118 Fetal heart auscultation with hand-held Doppler.

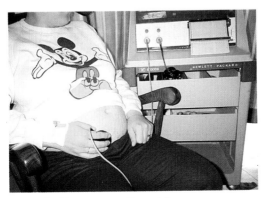

Fig. 119 Fetal heart rate recording technique.

Biophysical testing

Non-stress fetal heart rate (FHR) monitoring

There is a close association between an abnormal FHR pattern and an asphyxiated fetus. The normal FHR trace at term is dependent on the state of the fetus. A mature fetus will be quiet for about 30% of the time (very little movements and a 'flat' trace—little oscillation of the baseline and no accelerations), and active for about 70% of the time (repeated movements and an 'accelerative' or 'reactive' trace—wide oscillations of the baseline and many accelerations of 15 beats per min (bpm) or more). The presence of accelerations, a baseline rate of between 120–160 bpm and no decelerations (Fig. 120) is interpreted as reassuring of no evidence of asphyxia—in contrast to the fetus that is severely asphyxiated chronically (e.g. severe IUGR—Fig. 121) or acutely (e.g. placental haemorrhage—Fig. 122).

Biophysical profile scoring (BPS)

A more comprehensive assessment of the fetus at risk of asphyxia is provided by the BPS which records the presence of five biophysical variables: FHR pattern (non-stress test as above), fetal movements, fetal tone, fetal breathing and amniotic fluid volume. If four or five of these parameters are present in up to 40 min of recording then the risk of terminal fetal asphyxia is low.

Non-asphyxial causes of death

The biophysical methods of fetal assessment described above are valid for asphyxiated fetuses and probably those that are infected. Their value in other pathologies (e.g. metabolic) is not established.

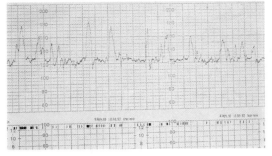

Fig. 120 Normal antepartum fetal heart rate recording at term.

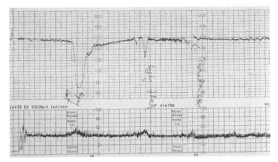

Fig. 121 Recording from asphyxiated growth retarded fetus.

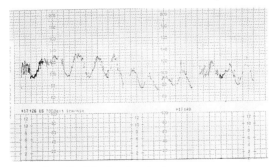

Fig. 122 Recording following abruptio placentae.

Doppler recording of blood flow

The absence of forward flow in diastoly in the umbilical arteries of a small-for-dates (SFD) fetus (Figs 123 & 124) is associated with an increased risk of IUGR, perinatal death, birth asphyxia, neonatal respiratory distress (and its complications) and necrotizing enterocolitis. Thus it may be of value in ascribing the degree of risk in the SFD fetus.

Kleihauer test

This detects fetal red blood cells (rbc) in maternal blood. Fetal rbc (containing haemoglobin-F) are less likely to haemolyse in alkaline pH than are maternal cells (containing haemoglobin-A) (Fig. 125). The test is used (i) after a potential sensitizing event in a rhesus-negative mother (p. 45) and (ii) to confirm a fetomaternal transfusion when there is a suspicion of concealed placental bleeding (p. 99).

Radiology

Radiological techniques can be used to measure the bony pelvis (pelvimetry) (see pp. 123–124) with, for example, a breech presentation at 37 weeks, suspected cephalopelvic disproportion, pelvic injury or disease and possible contraction (average anteroposterior diameters are: inlet 11.5 cm, midcavity 12.0 cm, outlet 12.5 cm). Use of pelvimetry has declined and its value is questionable except where a contracted pelvis is suspected. Where it is indicated, CT or MRI pelvimetry have now largely replaced X-rays. Plain X-rays are undertaken if there is a clinical indication (such as a chest X-ray for suspected pneumonia or abdominal X-ray for suspected intestinal obstruction) where the risks of missing the diagnosis outweigh the risks from the X-rays. Contrast studies are generally avoided in pregnancy with ultrasound being the mainstay of maternal renal examination. If an intravenous pyelogram is performed after delivery, it is advisable for this to be deferred for 3 months so that the physiological changes of pregnancy have resolved (Fig. 126).

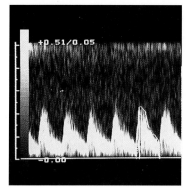

Fig. 123 Doppler recording from umbilical artery (normal).

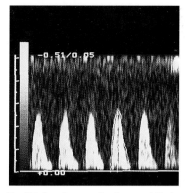

Fig. 124 Doppler recording from umbilical artery (absent end diastolic flow).

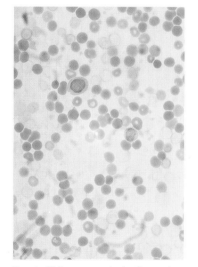

Fig. 125 Kleihauer test—fetal cells remain intact, maternal cells have haemolysed.

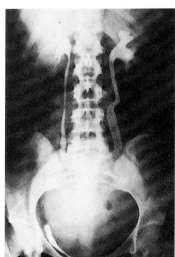

Fig. 126 Intravenous pyelogram—effects of pregnancy.

Premature rupture of membranes (PROM)

Definition/ incidence

Membrane rupture before uterine contractions. 10% of all pregnancies, 30% of preterm deliveries.

Risks

- Labour/delivery; risks to baby if preterm.
- Sepsis; this is the main risk at term.
- Effects of oligohydramnios: pulmonary hypoplasia (PROM before 26 weeks), cord compression, postural deformities.

Diagnosis

Liquor at introitus or in vagina (Fig. 127).

Management

General: Vigilance for infection until delivery (maternal temperature, pulse, FHR, culture of liquor or low vaginal swab and urine, uterine tenderness or contractions). Avoid vaginal examinations unless labour suspected. Value of prophylactic antibiotics is uncertain. Amniocentesis for microbiological examination if uncertainty about infection. Delivery is expedited if intrauterine infection suspected.

After 34 weeks: Induction after an interval.

Before 34 weeks: Do not stop spontaneous. labour. Give weekly dexamethasone to improve fetal surfactant production.

Preterm labour and delivery (<37 weeks)

Incidence

Approximately 5% of all deliveries.

Causes

Twins, fetal and uterine abnormality, placental bleeding, infection, incompetent cervix, PROM.

Management

Confirm diagnosis (uterine activity *plus* cervical changes). Search for a cause. If no contraindication (34 weeks or more, bleeding, abnormal fetus), administer i.v. tocolytics (e.g. salbutamol). Give dexamethasone to reduce risk of respiratory distress syndrome (RDS).

Neonatal complications

Include: RDS (Fig. 128), hypothermia, poor feeding, jaundice, hypoglycaemia, infection (Fig. 129).

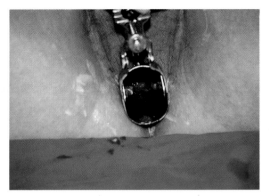

Fig. 127 Liquor in vagina seen through sterile speculum.

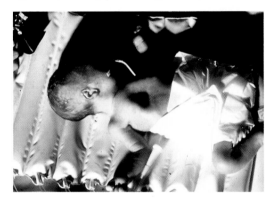

Fig. 128 Preterm newborn infant with respiratory distress.

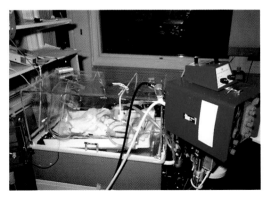

Fig. 129 Intensive care for the preterm infant (assisted ventilation, i.v. feeding, incubator to control temperature).

Onset

Definition

'The process of birth': characterized by regular contractions, effacement and dilatation of the cervix and descent of the presenting part.

Onset

When regular uterine contractions and cervical changes begin. Diagnosis is not always easy (Braxton Hicks contractions can be mistaken for labour; cervical effacement can predate dilatation by several days).

Diagnosis

- Palpation of 'painful' regular contractions (Fig. 130), with a frequency of 1+ in 5 min, a duration of 20+ s.
- Evidence of cervical effacement and/or dilatation (Fig. 131).

The onset of labour is often associated with a 'show'—the passage vaginally of a blood-stained mucus plug from the cervix (Fig. 132). Membrane rupture is not necessary for the diagnosis of labour. It only precedes labour in about 10% of cases.

First stage

Definition

'From the onset of labour to full dilatation of the cervix.'
- *Latent phase*: 'from the onset of labour to when the cervix is about 3 cm dilated and fully effaced'. Mean length (±SD) is 9 (±6) h in primigravidae and 5 (±4) h in multigravidae.
- *Active phase*: 'dilatation of the cervix from 3 cm'. The mean length (±SD) is 5 (±3.5) h in primigravidae and 2 (±1.5) h in multigravidae.

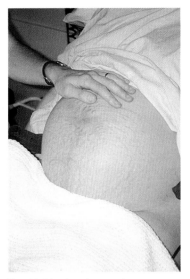

Fig. 130 Palpation of contraction.

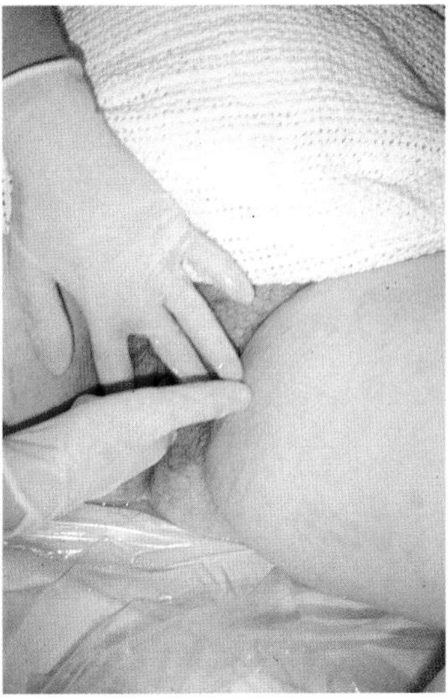

Vaginal examination image

Fig. 131 Vaginal examination.

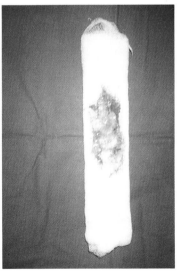

Fig. 132 'Show'.

Induction

Indications

The decision to end a pregnancy is because the infant will be safer if delivered, or the risk to the maternal health of continuing with the pregnancy outweighs the risk to the baby of delivery.

If the risk of labour is unacceptable, then delivery should be by caesarean section. In other cases labour can be induced. Maternal indications may include hypertension, diabetes and cardiac disease. Fetal indications may include growth retardation, multiple pregnancy and premature rupture of the membranes at term.

Contra-indications

- *Absolute*: include a fetal lie that is not longitudinal and an insuperable obstruction to vaginal delivery, previous upper segment caesarean section ('classical') (see p. 117) or uterine rupture.
- *Extreme caution*: induction with grand multiparity, previous uterine scar.

Methods

- Membrane rupture (amniotomy) with an amnihook (Fig. 133). This may have to be coupled with an i.v. infusion of an oxytocic agent.
- Most inductions, however, are undertaken with prostaglandin-E_2 in many formulations: the majority of inductions use vaginal tablets or pessaries, or gel (Fig. 134). Vaginal delivery of a dead fetus or a fetus with a lethal malformation is sometimes undertaken using extra-amniotic preparations administered via an endocervical catheter.

Complications

Iatrogenic prematurity, hyperstimulation (Fig. 135), infection, or failed induction. Large doses of synthetic oxytocin can produce neonatal jaundice and water intoxication of mother and baby.

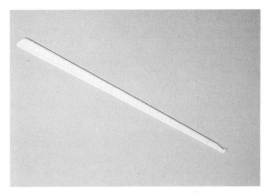

Fig. 133 Amnihook.

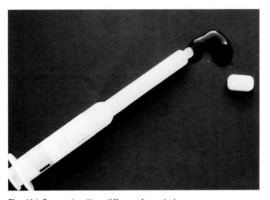

Fig. 134 Prostaglandins; different formulations.

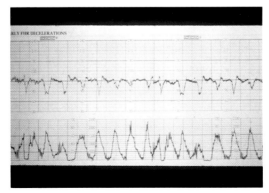

Fig. 135 Uterine hyperstimulation (excessively frequent contractions and fetal heart rate decelerations).

Management

Preparation

Classes organized by midwives are available in most areas. Visits to hospital are usually arranged.

General principles

Everyone involved in the birth of a child should be concerned with the safety and health of the mother and baby, and strive to make the birth a satisfying experience for all concerned.

In many countries overall conduct is the responsibility of a midwife alone or with reference to a general practitioner. An obstetrician need only be involved in those labours where problems are present (e.g. fetal distress, poor progress in labour, maternal disease). However, in other countries (e.g. North America) the great majority of deliveries are conducted by obstetricians.

Monitoring

Labour should be a normal event and management incorporates a programme of surveillance monitoring which confirms that it remains normal. There are three components of this monitoring, summarized on the partogram.

- *Fetal condition* (Fig. 136): a record of the fetal heart rate recorded every quarter hour, colour of liquor drained vaginally and the degree of caput and/or moulding judged from vaginal examinations performed every 3–4 h.
- *Progress of labour* (Fig. 137): record of the descent of the head (assessed abdominally in fifths, and vaginally with respect to the ischial spines), the dilatation of the cervix on regular vaginal examinations, the strength and frequency of contractions and drugs given to augment/induce labour.
- *Maternal condition* (Fig. 138): general well-being, pulse and blood pressure every half hour, temperature every 4 h and fluid balance are recorded. All drugs given are noted. Urine passed is tested for glucose, protein and ketones.

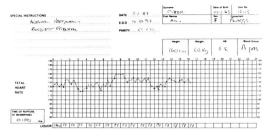

Fig. 136 Partogram—fetal section.

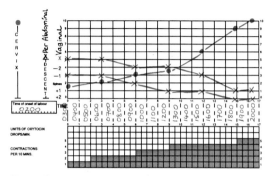

Fig. 137 Partogram—progress section.

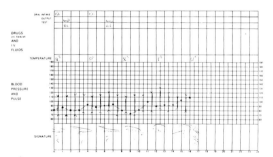

Fig. 138 Partogram—maternal section.

Fetal monitoring

Liquor

Normally the liquor is clear. Passage of meconium (Fig. 139) may be due to hypoxia and is an indication for continuous fetal heart rate (FHR) monitoring. Innocent causes are post-dates fetus and breech presentation. When meconium is present the baby is also at risk of meconium aspiration and requires expert care at birth. Mild blood staining may be just a 'show'. Heavier bleeding may be due to placental abruption, placenta praevia or vasa praevia (see pp. 101–104).

Moulding/caput

Severe degrees are significant, especially with poor progress of the labour (pp. 87–90) which may reflect cephalopelvic disproportion.

FHR monitoring

Routine: the fetal heart is normally recorded intermittently (every 15 min). The baseline should be between 110–150 bpm. Continuous FHR monitoring should be employed with pregnancies with an increased risk of intrapartum hypoxia, e.g. growth retardation, prematurity, breech presentation, multiple pregnancy, epidural analgesia, induced or augmented labour, diabetes, hypertension, bleeding, rhesus disease, auscultated FHR abnormalities, or meconium staining.

Continuous: the methods are external Doppler recording (Fig. 140) or electrically triggered signals with a fetal skin electrode (Fig. 141). Inherent risks of skin electrodes (see p. 131) make an external transducer preferable (provided a good quality recording is obtained). ➡

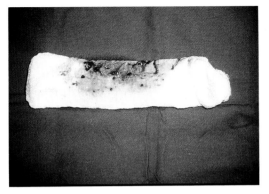

Fig. 139 Meconium.

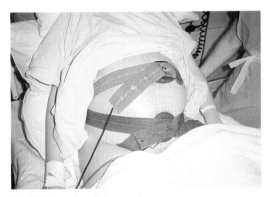

Fig. 140 External cardiotocography.

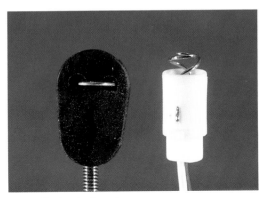

Fig. 141 Fetal scalp electrodes.

FHR monitoring

Screening procedure for fetal hypoxia. Fetal hypoxia causes a rise of PCO$_2$, a respiratory acidosis and an accumulation of lactate due to anaerobic glycolysis. The fetal blood pH falls. Interpretation of the significance of an FHR abnormality depends on the subsequent estimation of fetal pH by fetal blood sampling (FBS) (p. 85).

Fetal heart rates

Normal pattern (Fig. 142):   baseline rate 110–150 bpm, variation of 5 or more bpm, no decelerations, acceleration with fetal movements or contractions.

Loss of baseline/short term variability (<5 bpm):   can be seen with fetal hypoxia (FBS indicated if prolonged), or maternal drug therapy (e.g. pethidine).

Baseline bradycardia (<110 bpm):   low baselines (105–110 bpm) may be normal if postdates. Lower rates, especially if accompanied by other adverse features, are indications for FBS.

Fetal tachycardia: (baseline rate >150 bpm, no accelerations) may be due to hypoxia thus FBS advisable. Also seen with maternal pyrexia.

Decelerations:
- *early* (Fig. 143): begins with contraction and returns to baseline by end of contraction; commonly due to change of pressure on fetal head (engagement, full dilatation) (5% risk of low pH)
- *variable* (Fig. 144): in timing with respect to contraction, depth and duration; often due to cord compression (25% risk of low pH)
- *late* (Fig. 145): large deceleration of FHR after the contraction; commonly due to placental insufficiency (50% risk of low pH).

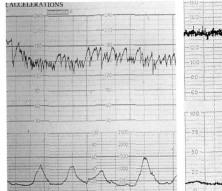

Fig. 142 Normal cardiotocograph.

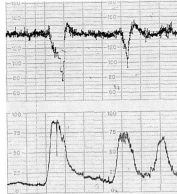

Fig. 143 Early decelerations.

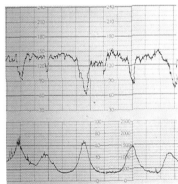

Fig. 144 Variable decelerations.

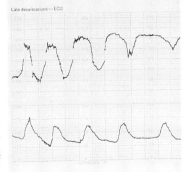

Fig. 145 Late decelerations.

Fetal blood sampling (FBS)

With an abnormal FHR trace, turn the mother on her left side, give oxygen by face mask, stop Syntocinon infusion (if present) and take FBS if abnormality persists.

Aim

To discover whether an abnormal FHR is due to fetal hypoxia and prevent severe asphyxia (white, apnoeic, hypotonic, bradycardic baby showing paucity of movement).

Equipment

pH meter, a cold light source, ethyl chloride spray, antiseptic lotions and cream, silicone jelly, small magnet with iron 'fleas' to stir the sample, and a pre-packed tray (Fig. 146) (amnioscopes, long instruments, 2 mm guarded blade, heparinized capillary tubes and swabs).

Procedure

The mother is placed in the left lateral position or in the lithotomy position with some lateral tilt, cleaned and gowned. An appropriately sized amnioscope is inserted through the cervix up against the fetal scalp (or buttocks if breech). The light source is attached. The fetal scalp is cleaned and a smear of silicone jelly applied. An assistant sprays the fetal scalp for 10 s to produce hyperaemia. The scalp is stabbed once with the guarded blade (Fig. 147) A continuous column of blood (10–30 µl), free of air bubbles, is collected in the capillary tube (Fig. 148). Pressure is applied to the fetal scalp to secure haemostasis.

Interpretation

pH > 7.25 is normal; pH 7.20–7.25 is borderline, (repeat within 30 min); pH < 7.20 is abnormal and delivery should be expedited.

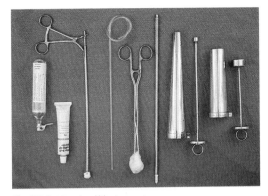

Fig. 146 Fetal scalp pH instruments.

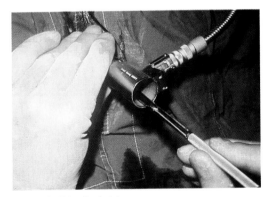

Fig. 147 Stabbing fetal scalp.

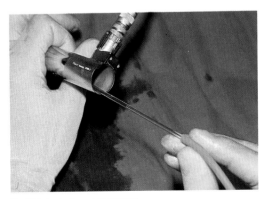

Fig. 148 Aspiration of fetal blood.

Progress

Normal progress in the first stage of labour

This has already been described (pp. 75–79) (Fig. 149). In primigravidae, delivery can be expected within 8 h of the diagnosis of labour and should be achieved within 12 h.

Causes

Delay in the first stage of labour

- Inefficient uterine action (IUA).
- Cephalopelvic disproportion (CPD) (either 'relative' due to occipitoposterior position (OPP) of fetal head, or 'absolute' due to large fetus and/or small maternal pelvis).

Patterns

- Slow progress (Fig. 150) which is more commonly, although not always, found with IUA.
- Secondary arrest (Fig. 151) which is more commonly, although not always, found with CPD.

Management

What is the cause of the delay? Is there evidence of CPD (e.g. short mother, large baby, late engagement of fetal head, OPP)? Is there clinical evidence of IUA?

If it is possible that the cause is IUA and potentially correctable then:

- correct any ketosis/dehydration with oral or i.v. fluids
- rupture the membranes—if still intact
- if these measures are not successful then augmentation of labour should be considered (see p. 89).
- evaluation of effect of management (see p. 89).

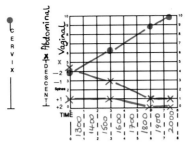

Fig. 149 Partogram—normal progress.

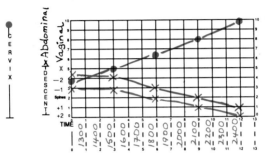

Fig. 150 Slow progress.

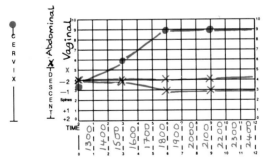

Fig. 151 Secondary arrest.

Augmentation of labour (see also p. 87).

The normal method is with a Syntocinon infusion (start at 2 mU/min and double every 20 min to a maximum of 32 mU/min until progress is achieved). Augmentation in a multiparous mother should only be undertaken after careful consideration by an experienced obstetrician (due to greater risk of uterine rupture). The use of an intrauterine pressure catheter (IUPC) (see below) may permit a more objective augmentation policy in certain cases.

Evaluation of management of delay

Once delay has been recognized and a management plan (p. 87) implemented, the effect of the management on the progress of labour is critically reviewed after 2–3 h. If the rate of progress has not been improved then caesarean section may have to be performed.

Contractions

Manual palpation is normally used to evaluate uterine activity. It is not a direct method. The presence of uterine activity in a poorly progressing labour does not necessarily mean the contractions are effective. An IUPC measures pressure directly (Figs 152, 153 & 154). Indications for use of this invasive procedure include management of augmented labour with possible CPD or a uterine scar. Between contractions the intrauterine pressure is usually <10 mmHg and at the peak of effective contractions, about 50 mmHg.

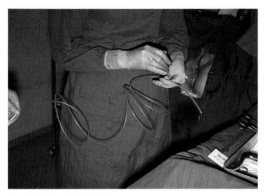

Fig. 152 Water-filled IUPC.

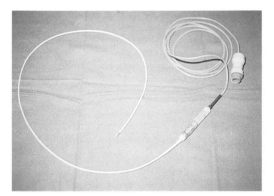

Fig. 153 Gaeltec IUPC.

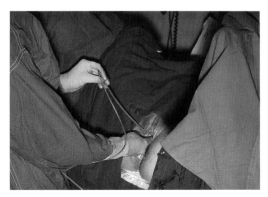

Fig. 154 Insertion IUPC.

General maternal condition

As far as possible, labour should be safe for both mother and baby and also an emotionally rewarding experience. Mobility should be encouraged during the latent phase of labour (Fig. 155).

Analgesia

The mother should decide whether she wants pain relief in labour, although the availability may vary. Ambulation (Fig. 155) and the presence of a supportive partner (Fig. 156) are helpful.

Psychological/relaxation methods may help. Antenatal education is an integral part of the process.

Inhalational agents: nitrous oxide (50%) and oxygen (50%) as Entonox (Fig. 156) are used by the mother often towards the end of the first stage and during the early part of the second stage. Longer administration is not practical. They are effective and safe for mother and baby.

Transcutaneous nerve stimulator (Fig. 157): this is usually only effective in early labour and with relatively mild contractions.

Opiates: intramuscular pethidine (meperidine) (50–150 mg) with or without a phenothiazine is the most widely used method of pain relief in Britain. The advantages of opiates are ease of administration, rapid effect, low incidence of serious side-effects and antagonists are available. Self-administration of intravenous pethidine by the mother is an alternative approach. The disadvantages include inadequate analgesia in 40% and vomiting is common. Neonatal respiratory depression can occur if the administration to delivery interval is <2 h. However, the effect is reversible with naloxone.

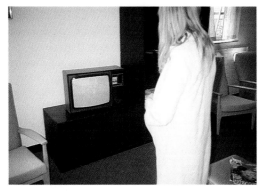

Fig. 155 Ambulation.

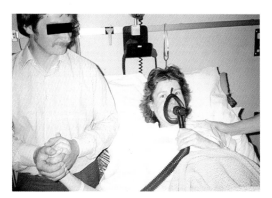

Fig. 156 Entonox and partner.

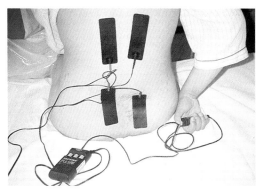

Fig. 157 Transcutaneous nerve stimulator.

Epidural analgesia

This is the most effective analgesic method, but experience in its use is essential.

Indications

On request, IUA, OPP, prolonged labour, breech presentation, multiple pregnancy, preterm labour, forceps delivery, hypertension, maternal distress/exhaustion.

Contra-indications

Lack of experienced personnel, infection at insertion site, spinal abnormalities, coagulation abnormalities, hypovolaemia. Careful monitoring is necessary with a previous caesarean section scar.

Complications

Dural puncture (headache), total spinal block (loss of sensory and motor function, unconsciousness, hypotension, apnoea), hypotension (due to caval compression, reduced venous return and cardiac output, and pooled blood in splanchnic bed), motor paralysis, urinary retention, toxic reactions and, rarely, an aseptic meningitis.

Management

The materials used are prepacked (Fig. 158). Insertion is in the left lateral or upright positions (Figs 159 & 160). The tip of the cannula lies in the epidural (extradural) space. Externally, the cannula is strapped up over the back and shoulder for ease of access (Fig. 161) with a bacterial filter attached.

An i.v. infusion of Hartmann's solution is first established to correct any possible hypotension (0.5%). Bupivacaine alone (repeated injections or as an infusion for continuous analgesia) or with opiates are the drugs commonly used. The dose is tailored to the patient. BP, respirations and FHR (continuous) are carefully monitored. The aim is to 'block'/anaesthetize T10–L1. An epidural or a single subarachnoid ('spinal') injection can provide regional analgesia for procedures such as manual removal of placenta or caesarean section.

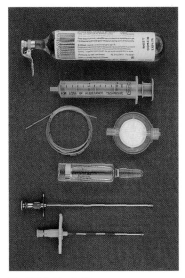

Fig. 158 Epidural—kit.

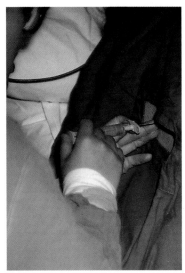

Fig. 159 Epidural—insertion (a).

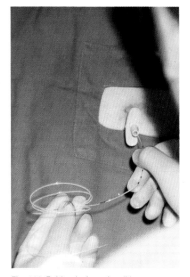

Fig. 160 Epidural—insertion (b).

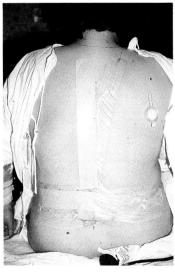

Fig. 161 Epidural—in use.

Second stage

From full dilatation of the cervix to delivery of the baby. Average duration is 40 min in primigravidae and 20 min in multiparae.

Propulsive: from full dilatation to the presenting part reaching the pelvic floor.

Expulsive: from then until the birth of the baby. The mother wishes to push or 'bear down' and the perineum is distended.

A mother should not normally be encouraged to push until the head is visible and/or the perineum is distended (Fig. 162). The decision to perform an episiotomy requires considerable experience and judgement (see also pp. 105–108). The aim of an episiotomy is to deliver the fetal head avoiding severe perineal tear. However, not all mothers will experience a severe perineal tear and certainly most multiparae will be able to have a delivery with an intact perineum. Primigravidae also may be able to avoid an episiotomy ('episiotomy for all primigravidae' should be discouraged).

If episiotomy is necessary then the perineum initially is infiltrated with 10 ml 1% lignocaine as it is distended (Fig. 163). The episiotomy (extending from the fourchette, posterolaterally, Fig. 164) is performed during a contraction when the perineum is maximally distended. The delivery of the fetal head (crowning) is controlled with the left hand on the vertex and the right hand applying a pad to the perineum (Fig. 165). Some advocate mid-line episiotomies though these have a higher incidence of anal sphincter and rectal damage. ➡

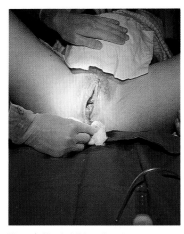

Fig. 162 Head visible at introitus.

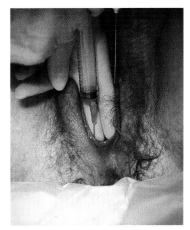

Fig. 163 Infiltration of perineum with local anaesthetic.

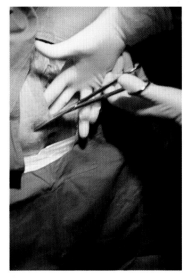

Fig. 164 Episiotomy.

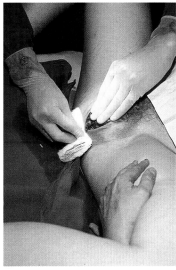

Fig. 165 Crowning of head.

The left hand (Fig. 166) prevents too rapid a delivery and decompression of the fetal head (especially important in the preterm infant). The right hand (Fig. 166) prevents uncontrolled tearing of the perineum. Once the head is delivered the face is wiped with a clean swab.

A hand is inserted to check for the presence of the cord around the baby's neck (Fig. 167). If found, it is either clamped and cut or pulled over the head.

Whilst the head is on the perineum it usually rotates to realign with the axis of the shoulders. The mother pushes again and, with the hands placed over the baby's parietal eminences, gentle traction is applied posteriorly to encourage the delivery of the anterior shoulder (Fig. 168).

Anterior traction is then applied and the posterior shoulder and the body are delivered. An intramuscular injection of an oxytocic agent is given with the delivery of the anterior shoulder (p. 99). Once the baby is delivered the cord is double-clamped and cut. The baby is dried and wrapped (Fig. 169), checked to ensure that he or she is breathing normally and handed to the mother. The baby will later be cleaned, dressed and placed in a cot.

Apgar score is traditionally used to record the condition of the baby at birth (at 1, 5 and 10 min).

Sign	Score = 0	Score = 1	Score = 2
Heart rate	Absent	<100/min	>100/min
Respiratory effort	Absent	Weak/irregular	Good/crying
Muscle tone	Flaccid	Flexion of extremities	Well flexed
Reflex irritability	None	Grimace	Cough/sneeze
Colour	White	Blue	Pink

A score of 7–10 is normal

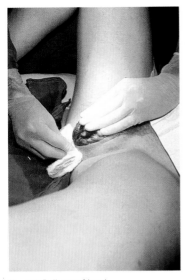

Fig. 166 Delivery of head.

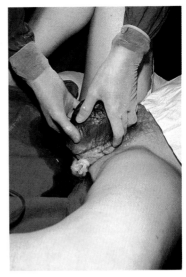

Fig. 167 Check for cord.

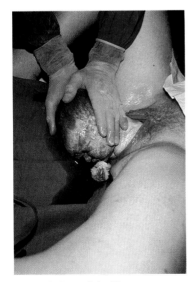

Fig. 168 Delivery of shoulders.

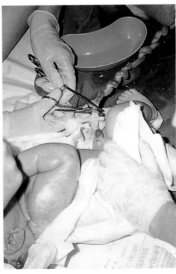

Fig. 169 Drying and wrapping baby and clamping cord.

Third stage

Definition

This begins after delivery of the baby and ends when the placenta is delivered.

Management

- *Active* (most common form in UK): administration of an oxytocic agent (intramuscular (i.m.) Syntometrine containing 5 units Syntocinon and 0.5 mg ergometrine or i.m. Syntocinon 10 units) with the delivery of the anterior shoulder (p. 97); clamping and cutting the cord (Fig. 169, p. 98) and delivery of the placenta once there are signs of separation (contraction of the uterus, a gush of blood (Fig. 170) and descent/lengthening of the cord). The placenta and membranes are delivered by controlled cord traction (Figs 171 & 172).
- *Passive:* no oxytocic agent, no cord clamping and waiting for the spontaneous delivery of the placenta. Higher incidence of primary postpartum haemorrhage.

Primary postpartum haemorrhage

Incidence

Occurs in 5% of births.

Definition

'The loss of 500 ml of blood or more within 24 h of delivery.'

Causes

Causes include hypotonic uterus (caused by wholly or partially retained placenta, multiple pregnancy, large baby, hydramnios, lax uterus associated with high parity); trauma (such as uterine rupture, cervical or vaginal lacerations) and clotting disorder. The two principles of management are resuscitation measures, and to identify and treat the cause.

Uterine atony is treated by intravenous oxytocics or prostaglandins (administered intramuscularly or intramyometrially). An examination under anaesthetic may be necessary if the cause is uncertain. Internal iliac artery ligation or hysterectomy may be necessary on rare occasions.

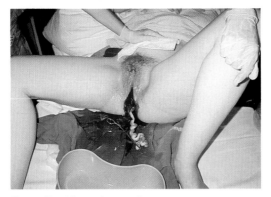

Fig. 170 Blood flow and contraction.

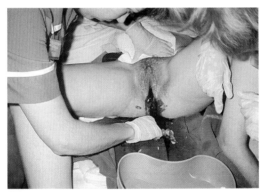

Fig. 171 Controlled cord traction.

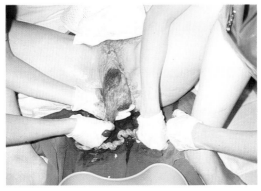

Fig. 172 Delivery of placenta.

Early development

Implantation of the blastocyst occurs approximately 6 or 7 days following fertilization. The solid inner cell mass forms the fetus, whilst the cyst wall becomes the trophoblast.

The trophoblast differentiates into an inner layer (cytotrophoblast) and an outer layer (syncytiotrophoblast). The endometrium becomes decidua (Fig. 173).

By the 14th day the trophoblast has developed into chorionic villi with a central core of mesenchyme. The villi eventually disappear from the surface of the blastocyst except in the area adjacent to the uterus; this will form the placenta. During the second trimester, the syncytiotrophoblast degenerates and the normal haemochorial circulation is formed.

Functions of the placenta

These are respiratory (gas exchange), nutritional (food and waste products), protein production (oestrogen, progesterone, hCG, human placental lactogen and other placental proteins).

Pathology

Morbid adherence (placenta accreta) (Fig. 174): the placenta implants into the myometrium. It is more common when the placenta implants over a uterine scar. It is a cause of retained placenta and post-partum haemorrhage (PPH). Uncontrollable haemorrhaging may necessitate hysterectomy.

Infection (chorioamnionitis) (Fig. 175): associated with prolonged rupture of the membranes and fetal death.

Succenturiate lobe (Fig. 176, p. 104): the placenta is in two parts linked by communicating vessels.

Velamentous insertion: cord divides and crosses the membranes to the placenta.

Multiple pregnancy (Fig. 177, p. 104): there can be a pathological communication.

Antepartum haemorrhage (see p. 103).

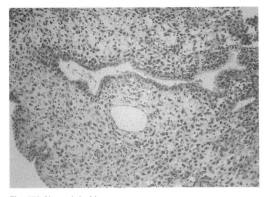

Fig. 173 Normal decidua.

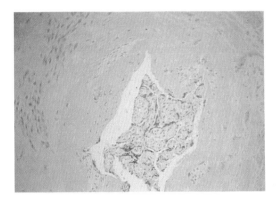

Fig. 174 Placenta accreta (placenta in uterine blood vessel).

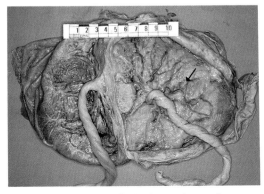

Fig. 175 Amnionitis in one of twin placentas (arrowed).

Antepartum haemorrhage

'Bleeding from the genital tract from 24 weeks and before delivery of the baby'.

- *Placenta praevia*: bleeding from placenta encroaching into the lower uterine segment. Usually painless.
- *Placental abruption*: bleeding from a normally situated placenta. Usually painful. Amount of blood passed vaginally can vary.
- *Vasa praevia*: bleeding from ruptured vessel in membranes. Often follows amniotomy with velamentous insertion or succenturiate lobe (Fig. 176).
- *'Show'*: at the onset of labour.
- *Bleeding from other sites* (e.g. cervix).

- Assess blood loss and resuscitate.
- The fetal condition should be assessed.
- Establish cause. A vaginal examination should be avoided until the placental site is known.
- If the bleeding ceases and the fetus is healthy, a placenta praevia is managed as in-patient (close to emergency caesarean section and blood transfusion available promptly), other causes are managed as out-patients.
- If the bleeding continues the delivery should be expedited, the route chosen (vaginal or abdominal) depending on the amount of bleeding, gestation and fetal health.

The value of placental examination after delivery is variable: it is unhelpful in, for example, IUGR and pre-eclampsia but useful to find a lost IUCD (Fig. 178), to diagnose chorioamnionitis, to identify a pathological vascular communication in multiple pregnancy, and to diagnose monochorionic twins.

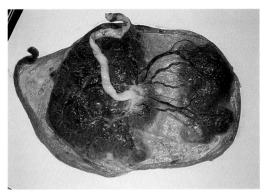

Fig. 176 Succenturiate lobe.

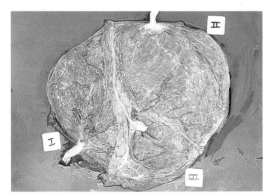

Fig. 177 Triplet placentae.

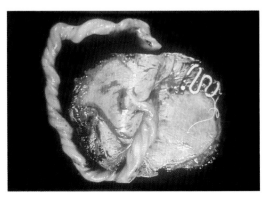

Fig. 178 Intrauterine contraceptive device in placenta.

Indications for episiotomy

The decision to perform an episiotomy should never be 'routine', but rather a matter for experienced clinical judgement. Possible indications include:

- avoidance of inevitable severe perineal tear
- fetal distress late in second stage
- most forceps deliveries (to avoid tears)
- breech delivery.

The episiotomy (posterolateral) should be performed with sharp scissors at the correct time (too early results in unnecessary blood loss, while too late may end with a perineal tear anyway), with adequate local or regional (epidural or spinal block) analgesia and repaired properly as quickly as possible after delivery.

Technique

The patient is placed in the lithotomy position and the vulva and perineum cleaned and gowned. Lighting and the field of view should be adequate. There should be adequate analgesia using local anaesthetic (Fig. 179) or regional analgesia.

Vaginal skin: the apex of the vaginal incision must be clearly identified (Fig. 180). The vaginal skin is repaired with a continuous suture of either chromic catgut or polyglycolic acid, starting just above the apex of the incision (Fig. 181). Care must be taken to ensure an even apposition of the vaginal skin edges. The suture is tied at the level of the carunculae myritiformes (remnants of the hymen).

Perineal tissues: on completion of the vaginal suturing the defect in the perineum should be approximately elliptical (Fig. 182). The deep tissues of the perineum are repaired with interrupted sutures of either chromic catgut or polyglycolic acid. ➡

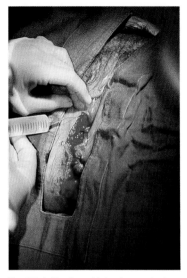

Fig. 179 Infiltration with local anaesthetic.

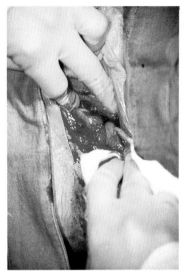

Fig. 180 Inspection of apex of vaginal incision.

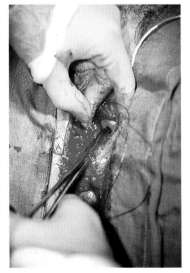

Fig. 181 Vaginal suture.

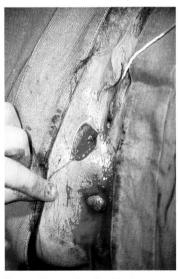

Fig. 182 Unsutured perineal body.

The perineal body sutures (Fig. 183) are inserted with care to avoid penetration of the rectum and at right angles to the axis of the defect.

Perineal skin: the perineal skin is repaired with either chromic catgut or polyglycolic acid sutures. Interrupted sutures (Fig. 184) or a subcuticular technique may be used. After the repair has been completed a vaginal examination is performed (Fig. 185) to check that no swabs have been left in the vagina and that there is no remaining defect or haematoma. Finally, a rectal examination is performed to confirm that no sutures have penetrated the rectal mucosa (Fig. 186).

Aftercare
Adequate analgesia should be offered to the mother, both systemic (oral analgesics) and topical (ice-packs, haemalis water).

Perineal tears

First degree (skin only) and *second degree* (skin and perineal body) *perineal tears* are managed and repaired in the same way.

Third/fourth degree tear is a tear which extends to include the anal sphincter (third degree) and/or rectum (fourth degree). It is repaired in theatre under general or regional anaesthesia by an experienced obstetrician. The rectum and anus are first repaired with interrupted chromic catgut sutures (knots in rectal lumen) and then the edges of the sphincter are apposed and sutured. The residual second degree tear is repaired separately afterwards. The mother is given a high fibre diet, aperient and antibiotics afterwards. The time for recovery/healing of an episiotomy scar is longer than many expect. For example, as many as 20% of women will have a tender scar 6 weeks after the delivery.

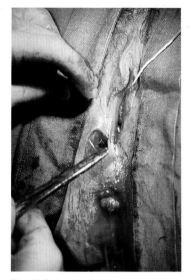

Fig. 183 Perineal body suture.

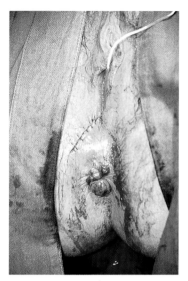

Fig. 184 Sutured skin.

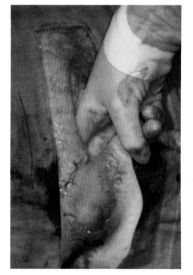

Fig. 185 Vaginal examination.

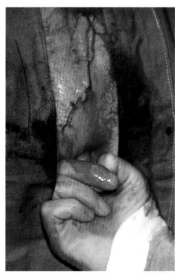

Fig. 186 Rectal examination.

Prerequisites

- A valid indication must exist (see below).
- Suitable presentation.
- No cephalopelvic disproportion and no excessive moulding.
- Engaged head and ideally no fetal head palpable per abdomen.
- Known position of the fetal head.
- Full dilatation of the cervix.
- Adequate analgesia.
- Empty bladder.
- Adequate uterine contractions.

These requirements apply to use of the ventouse (p. 113), except that it may be used before full cervical dilatation (9 cm or more).

Indications

- Maternal conditions where prolonged expulsive efforts may be contraindicated, e.g. cardiac disease, hypertension, dural puncture.
- Fetal distress in the second stage.
- Cord prolapse in the second stage.
- Poor progress in the second stage due to maternal exhaustion or occipitoposterior position.

Types

Non-rotational: suitable for occipito-anterior positions of the fetal head (A in Fig. 187). They have a cephalic curve and a pelvic curve (e.g. Rhodes', Wrigley's, Simpson's).

Rotational: suitable for transverse or occipito posterior positions (B in Fig. 187). They only have a cephalic curve (e.g. Kielland's).

Procedure

Non-rotational: after abdominal palpation, the mother is placed in the lithotomy position, cleaned, gowned and catheterized (Fig. 188). A vaginal examination is performed to confirm full dilatation; check the position and station, and assess pelvic capacity (Fig. 189). ➡

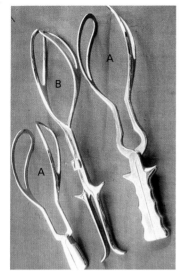

Fig. 187 Variation in forceps.

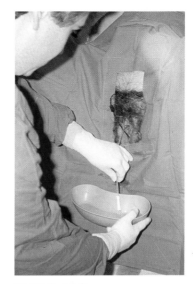

Fig. 188 Preparation.

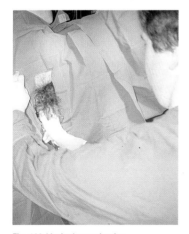

Fig. 189 Vaginal examination.

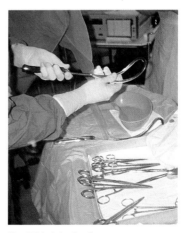

Fig. 190 Lubricating forceps.

Analgesia must be adequate: regional analgesia (e.g. epidural) or local anaesthetic with 1% lignocaine (pudendal and perineal blocks). The forceps blades are lubricated (Fig. 190, p. 110) and guided alongside the fetal head (left blade first) (Fig. 191). Traction is applied with a contraction and maternal effort (Fig. 192). An episiotomy is normally performed and the head delivered gently with protection of the perineum as for a normal delivery (Fig. 193). The forceps blades are removed (Fig. 194). The remainder of the delivery is as for a normal delivery (p. 97).

Definition of terms

Occipitoposterior delivery ('face to pubes'): in certain cases it may be preferable to deliver in the occipitoposterior position without rotation (e.g. deeply engaged head, or pelvis with narrow transverse diameter inhibiting rotation). This method of delivery requires great judgement, experience and skill.

Forceps for delivery of the head with a breech presentation: this method allows control of the delivery preventing intracranial trauma.

Forceps for delivery of low birth weight (LBW) infants: there is no evidence that elective forceps delivery of LBW infants confers any benefit on the baby.

Trial of forceps: this term refers to those cases where it is considered likely, although not totally certain, that vaginal delivery by forceps will be successful. A trial of forceps must be carried out by an experienced obstetrician in a theatre prepared for immediate caesarean section.

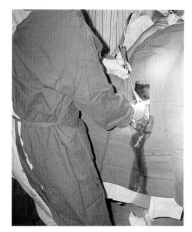

Fig. 191 Applying blade.

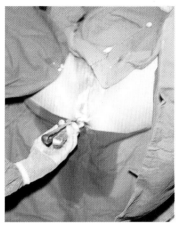

Fig. 192 Traction.

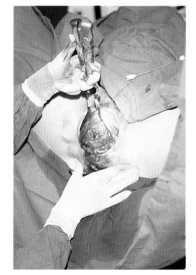

Fig. 193 Head crowning.

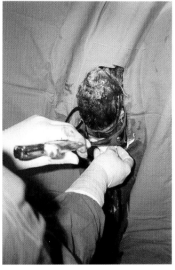

Fig. 194 Removal of forceps.

19 / Ventouse

Indications	Same as for forceps.
Instruments	Stainless steel or plastic cup, diameter varies (40 mm, 50 mm or 60 mm) with size of baby's head, and a chain and suction tube (Fig. 195).
Technique	A suitably sized cup is applied as near to the occiput as possible (to maintain flexion during traction) (Fig. 196) and a vacuum is created by means of a hand or electric pump (Fig. 197). The pressure is initially increased to 0.2 kg/cm^2 and having checked there is no vagina or cervix included under the rim the pressure is gradually increased to 0.8 kg/cm^2. With metal cups this pressure is increased gradually over 5–6 min; with plastic cups the increase can take place over 1–2 min. This draws the scalp into the cup in the shape of a chignon or bun. Traction is then applied to the chain coinciding with uterine contractions and maternal pushing and when the head passes through the introitus, the suction is released.
Complications	Fetal scalp abrasions (Fig. 221, p. 128) and cephalhaematomas (Fig. 220, p. 128) are common. Retinal haemorrhages, intracranial haemorrhage and scalp necrosis rarely occur. Fetal haemorrhage may result if the cup is applied following fetal blood sampling.
Advantages	The ventouse can be applied near to full dilatation, and used for either low cavity or midcavity extraction where rotation of the fetal head is required. For the latter indication, it is easier to learn than rotational forceps, requires less analgesia and carries less risk of maternal trauma.
Disadvantages	Delivery time is prolonged (and so some obstetricians consider the method is inappropriate if there is fetal distress); it is relatively inefficient in cases of malrotation. It cannot be used in cases of face presentation or in a breech delivery for delivering the head.

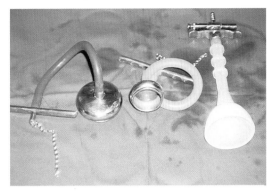

Fig. 195 Variety of cups.

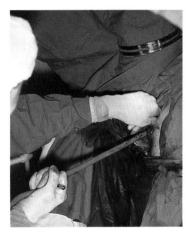

Fig. 196 Application of cups.

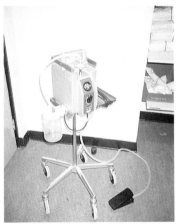

Fig. 197 Suction machine.

Incidence

Varies with policies of different centres. Currently 10–15% in UK and 20–25% in North America. May be elective (planned in advance) or an emergency. Maternal and perinatal mortality and morbidity are higher when the operation is an emergency.

Indications

Routine CS
- Previous CS for recurrent cause (e.g. small pelvis).
- Two or more previous CS.
- Breech presentation with small pelvis, and/or big baby, and/or footling presentation (the latter has an increased risk of cord prolapse).
- Placenta praevia.

Emergency CS
- Fetal distress (abnormal cardiotocography, acidosis, cord prolapse or abruption) before or during the first stage of labour.
- Obstructed labour (e.g. pelvic cyst/fibroid).
- Prolonged labour due to dysfunctional uterine activity or disproportion.
- Bleeding from placenta praevia.
- Preterm delivery with estimated fetal weight <1000 g but where there is prospect of viability (this is a controversial view).
- Preterm breech delivery where the estimated weight is 1000–1500 g.
- Delivery for maternal risk (e.g. uncontrollable HT, eclampsia) where prompt vaginal delivery is not feasible (usually preterm).

Technique up to incision

Following induction of general or regional (spinal) anaesthesia the patient is catheterized, and the abdomen is cleaned with antiseptic (Fig. 198) and draped with sterile towels. The abdomen is opened with either a lower transverse incision (Fig. 199) or a midline subumbilical incision. ➡

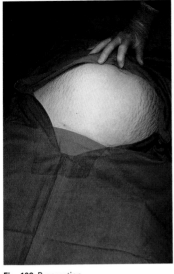

Fig. 198 Preparation.

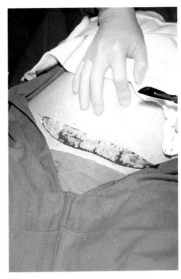

Fig. 199 Incision.

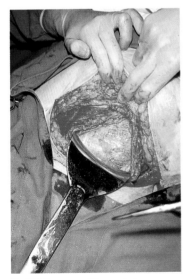

Fig. 200 Exposure of lower uterine segment.

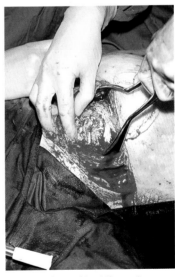

Fig. 201 Delivery of head (forceps).

Lower segment: this is the most common approach, used in 99% of cases. Uterovesical peritoneum is reflected (Fig. 200, p. 116) and the lower segment opened with a transverse incision. The risk of rupture in subsequent labour is low (about 0.1%).

Upper segment: this approach was used for several centuries, hence its description as 'classical'. Vertical incision is made in the upper segment of the uterus. Greater blood loss, higher risk of rupture in a subsequent labour (4–9%), and greater risk of bowel adhesions and postoperative ileus.

Note: the type of previous CS cannot be determined from the skin incision but rather is described by the incision made in the uterus.

- Transverse lie which cannot readily be converted to longitudinal (e.g. prolapsed arm).
- Certain uterine abnormalities, e.g. fibroids in the lower segment.
- Some cases of placenta praevia.
- For delivery of some low birth weight babies, particularly with oligohydramnios (poorly formed lower segment where delivery may be difficult and traumatic).
- Dense adhesions obscuring the lower segment.

The head is delivered either manually or with forceps (Figs 201, p. 116, & 202). Syntocinon is administered i.v. to the mother and the placenta delivered by cord traction (Fig. 203). The uterus is repaired in two layers of continuous absorbable sutures (Fig. 204). The abdomen is closed in layers (Fig. 205). Postoperative attention is paid to analgesia, physiotherapy, mobilization and assistance with feeding.

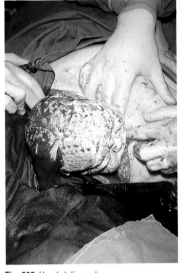

Fig. 202 Head delivered.

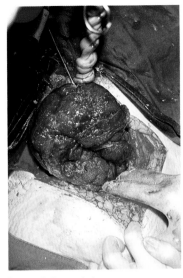

Fig. 203 Delivery of placenta.

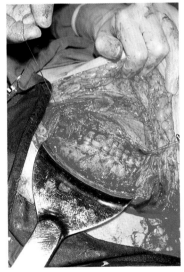

Fig. 204 Uterine repair.

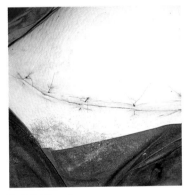

Fig. 205 Skin sutures.

Incidence	Difficult to determine (spontaneous abortion rate is higher, only one twin may be lost). The quoted incidence is 1 in 80 pregnancies although recent reports suggest 1 in 100. Higher-order multiples are much less common: triplets 1 in 80^2, quads 1 in 80^3 (higher incidence with modern techniques of assisted reproduction).
Types	*Monozygotic* (M–Z): results from fertilization of single ovum which divides into two embryos. Rarely share the same sac (1%) and very rarely are conjoined (Fig. 206). No racial or familial predisposition.
	Dizygotic (D–Z): results from multiple ovulation and fertilization. Strong familial and racial (Nigerian) predisposition. More frequent with greater maternal age, parity, height and obesity. The M–Z to D–Z ratio is 1:4.
Diagnosis	Large-for-dates, hyperemesis, a raised serum alphafetoprotein, or early HT. Ultrasound is the best method of diagnosis (Fig. 207). Clinical diagnosis is made by palpating more than two poles or detecting two fetal hearts.
General complications	With the exception of postmaturity, every complication of pregnancy is increased. Accounts for about 10% of perinatal deaths. Monochorionic twins have a much higher perinatal mortality as they run the risk of twin–twin transfusion syndrome.
Specific complications	*Twin–twin transfusion syndrome:* due to arteriovenous fistulae through which blood from one fetus drains via the placenta of the other (especially M–Z twins). The donor twin tends to be anaemic and growth-retarded with the recipient twin plethoric/polycythaemic and large-for-dates (Fig. 208).
	An extreme form results in the 'stuck twin syndrome' where there is anhydramnios (no amniotic fluid) around the donor twin resulting in

➡

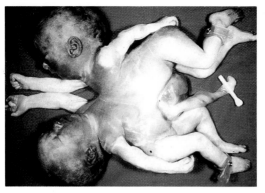

Fig. 206 Conjoined twins.

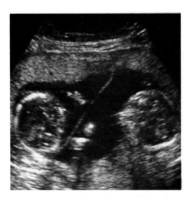

Fig. 207 Diagnosis by ultrasound (showing two heads and separating membrane).

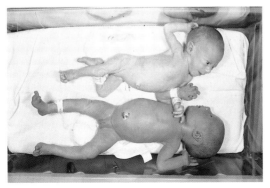

Fig. 208 Twin–twin transfusion.

that fetus being 'stuck' against the uterine wall. There is increasing hydramnios and hydrops in the recipient twin.

Monoamniotic twins are found in only 1% of all cases but can result in cord entanglement (Fig. 209) and twin entrapment during delivery.

Antenatal care

In addition to routine antenatal care:
- dietary supplementation of iron and folate
- more frequent antenatal checks
- detailed scan at 18 weeks (higher rate of fetal anomalies—Fig. 210)
- monthly growth scans thereafter (more often if discordant—Fig. 208, p. 120)
- vigilance for preterm labour (approximately 10% deliver <28 weeks and 30% deliver <37 weeks). Routine hospitalization is no longer performed.

Some obstetricians advocate elective induction at 38 weeks for maternal comfort and to prevent any complications.

Mode of delivery

Generally, the mode of delivery is vaginal. If the first twin is breech (10–20%) then the same criteria are applied as if it were a singleton breech (see pp. 123–126).

Labour and delivery

Continuously monitor both fetuses. Epidural block is the preferred analgesia. Delivery of the first twin is as for a singleton. Delay in delivery of the second twin carries an increased risk of asphyxia. A Syntocinon infusion should be ready (contractions tend to subside after delivery of the first baby). The abdomen is palpated to determine the lie and presentation of the second twin (Fig. 211). A transverse lie is converted to longitudinal either by external version, or by grasping a foot vaginally. With the next contraction the mother recommences pushing and membranes are ruptured. The vagina usually permits easy spontaneous or assisted delivery of the second twin. Two paediatricians and double resuscitation facilities should be available at delivery (Fig. 212). The zygosity can be determined at birth in 80% of twins (sex unlike, or single chorion).

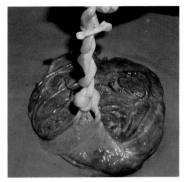

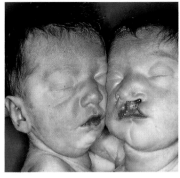

Fig. 209 Cord entanglement with monoamniotic twins.

Fig. 210 Risk of congenital anomaly.

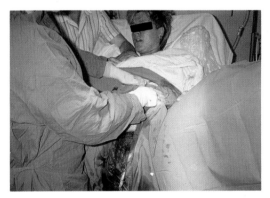

Fig. 211 Palpation of lie of second twin.

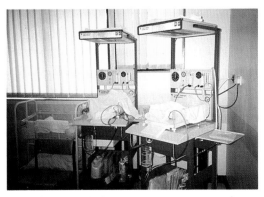

Fig. 212 Double paediatric resources.

Incidence	Decreases with advancing gestation (25% at 30 weeks and 3% at term).
Aetiology	• Uterine anomalies, e.g. fibroids, bicornuate uterus. • Fetal anomalies, e.g. hydrocephalus, anencephaly. • Multiple pregnancy. • Placenta praevia. In most cases no cause is identified.
Types	*Frank breech* (extended legs) is most common, then *flexed* and, least commonly, *footling*.
Management	Check for persistence of breech around 36 weeks. Pelvimetry may be performed but is no longer routine as its value is questioned (Figs 213 & 214). Pelvic diameters of less than 11.0 cm are generally considered inadequate for vaginal delivery. Scan to exclude hyperextension of the head (carrying a high risk of spinal cord injury) and gross abnormality, and to estimate fetal weight. Some consider a footling presentation to be an indication for caesarean section (risk of cord prolapse). The following should be considered: • *External cephalic version* (controversial): the breech is gently displaced upwards and the fetus encouraged to rotate by gentle pressure on either pole. It is more successful if the mother is given a tocolytic agent such as ritodrine or salbutamol. Rh-negative mothers should receive anti-D prophylaxis and the fetus should be monitored afterwards. • *Elective caesarean section*: increasingly used in the past decade, especially in the USA. • *Vaginal breech delivery* (see p. 129): if opted for, ultrasound is useful to estimate fetal weight (e.g. by measurement of abdominal circumference) at 38 weeks (Fig. 215), to exclude fetal anomaly and to diagnose a footling presentation.

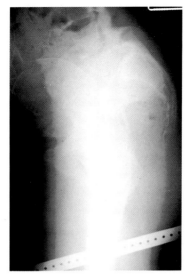

Fig. 213 X-ray pelvimetry. Posterior surface of symphysis pubis and anterior surface of sacrum are visible.

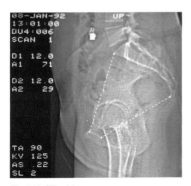

Fig. 214 CT-pelvimetry.

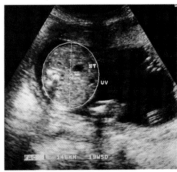

Fig. 215 US measurement of fetal abdominal circumference (weight estimation).

Delivery

Relative contraindications to vaginal delivery:
- estimated fetal weight below 1500 g or above 4000 g (risk of trauma/asphyxia)
- footling presentation (high incidence of cord prolapse)
- deflexion attitude.

Labour

Fetal heart rate monitored continuously. Slow progress and abnormal cardiotocography are commonly managed by CS, even in the second stage.

The use of augmentation with poor prognosis and taking a sample of blood from the fetal buttock for pH estimation are controversial measures.

Analgesia

Preferably epidural.

Delivery

Pushing is encouraged once the buttocks or feet (Fig. 216) are visible and a generous episiotomy is made with their delivery. Delivery to the umbilicus is by maternal effort alone. If the legs are extended their delivery is assisted by abduction and flexion at the knees (Fig. 217). The arms usually lie across the chest and maternal effort is sufficient to deliver the shoulders. If the arms are extended, a finger is passed over the shoulder to the antecubital fossa which is flexed and the arm brought down (Fig. 218). The fetus is either allowed to hang or delivered along the attendant's arm until the hairline is visible. Delivery of the head is controlled by laying the trunk astride an arm with a finger in the mouth and the other hand on the occiput (Mauriceau–Smellie–Veit manoeuvre), or by applying forceps after an assistant has lifted the feet (Fig. 219).

Complications

Asphyxia: cord compression or entrapment of head in incompletely dilated cervix.

Trauma: e.g. abdominal viscera, cervical spinal cord, brachial plexus, oedema and bruising of genitalia (Fig. 224, p. 130).

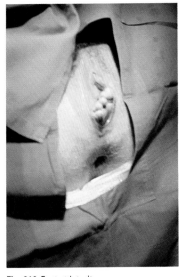

Fig. 216 Feet at introitus.

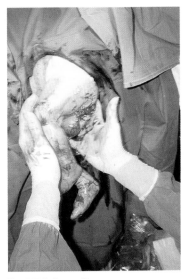

Fig. 217 Delivery of legs.

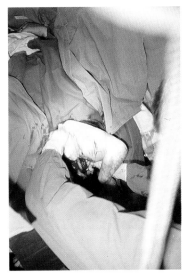

Fig. 218 Delivery of arms.

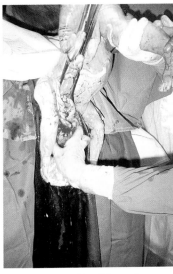

Fig. 219 Delivery of head (forceps).

Cephalhaematoma

Definition

Fluctuant mass loosely attached under the periosteum of cranial bones (commonly parietal) and not crossing the suture lines (Fig. 220).

Incidence

0.5–2.5% of vaginal deliveries.

Aetiology

May follow spontaneous delivery but more commonly follows forceps or ventouse (3%).

Course

May contribute to anaemia and jaundice. Usually resolves spontaneously over several weeks. Rarely calcification or infection occur.

Ventouse extraction

Scalp echymoses and artificial caput (chignon) always occur (Fig. 221). Chignon diminishes markedly in the first hour following delivery. Scalp abrasions (8%) take longer to resolve and necrosis is rare.

Forceps

Facial pressure marks (Fig. 222) are very common and disappear within hours. Abrasions may take some days to heal but rarely leave scars.

Facial palsy

Presents as asymmetry of the face on crying (Fig. 223).

Incidence

About 0.25% of births.

Aetiology

Compression of the facial nerve distal to the stylomastoid foramen during labour or delivery. More common following forceps but can follow normal delivery due to pressure on a maternal bony prominence or the fetus's own shoulder.

Management

Protect the eye which cannot be closed (lower motor neurone lesion).

Course

Most cases resolve within days.

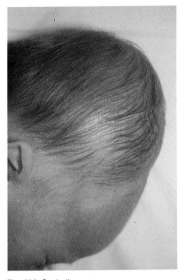

Fig. 220 Cephalhaematoma.

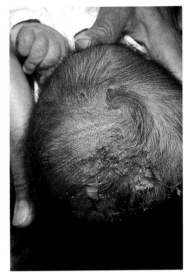

Fig. 221 Ventouse.

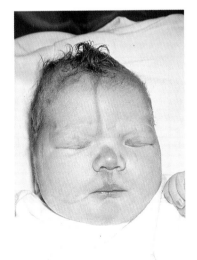

Fig. 222 Forceps mark.

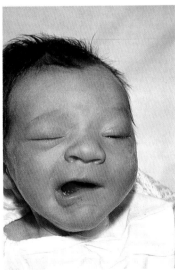

Fig. 223 Facial palsy.

Vaginal breech delivery

Vaginal breech delivery predisposes to certain types of injury including spinal cord lesions, peripheral nerve palsies, fractures of long bones and intracranial bleeding. Bruising of the genitalia (Fig. 224) is very common and resolves without long-term sequelae, although this is less certain in males.

Brachial plexus injuries

Types

Erb's palsy (97%) (lesion of C5, 6): internal rotation of arm with extension and adduction of hand; rarely phrenic nerve palsy (Fig. 225).

Klumpke's palsy (3%) (lesion of C8, T1): weakness of hand, rarely with Horner syndrome.

Aetiology

Traction on brachial plexus during delivery. More common after shoulder dystocia.

Prognosis

80% recover completely in 3–6 months. Occasionally there is severe permanent deficit resulting in a functionless short limb.

Tentorial tear (Fig. 226)

Aetiology

Hypoxia renders the brain oedematous and its supporting membranes rigid and prone to damage. Excessive moulding, prematurity, breech and forceps delivery are further predisposing factors.

Course

The infant is usually flaccid, pale and difficult to resuscitate at birth. Survivors have high incidence of neurological sequelae.

Injuries to intra-abdominal viscera

Tearing of the liver (Fig. 227) or spleen may follow breech delivery and is avoided by minimizing handling. Intraperitoneal haemorrhage results in shock and anaemia, and sometimes blood in the scrotum. Urgent laparotomy may be necessary.

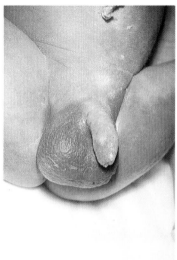

Fig. 224 Bruised genitalia.

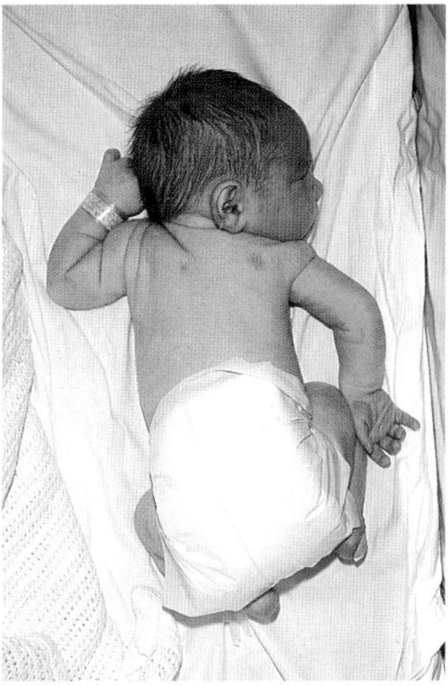

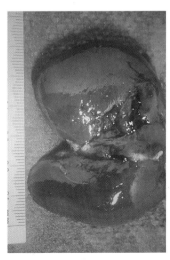

Fig. 225 Erb's palsy.

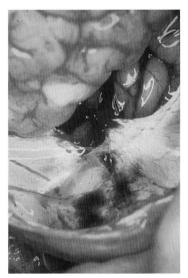

Fig. 226 Tentorial tear.

Fig. 227 Ruptured liver.

Injuries associated with fetal monitoring

A scalp abscess at the site of electrode application occurs in 0.5–5%. These usually resolve spontaneously with a small minority requiring surgical drainage and antibiotics. Removal of a piece of scalp (Figs 228 & 229) may occur when the electrode is pulled off at delivery. Fortunately, plastic surgical repair gives a good result.

Subconjunctival haemorrhages

These may be found following vaginal birth in both infant (Fig. 230) and mother (Fig. 237, p. 136). They resolve spontaneously and do not require any special management.

Injuries associated with caesarean section

All of the injuries mentioned in association with vaginal delivery have also been reported after caesarean section. Although widely regarded as a safer mode delivery of the infant by this route can occasionally be as difficult and traumatic as a vaginal delivery. Laceration of the fetus is only likely to occur at caesarean section and often involves the face (Fig. 231). This may result in an unsightly scar and may need treatment in the form of plastic surgery.

With such injuries it is advisable to show them to the parents, give a full explanation and answer any questions. Some advocate keeping a photographic record of the injury. Paediatric follow-up and review is advisable especially with facial injuries.

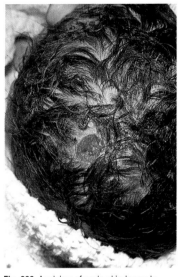

Fig. 228 Avulsion of scalp skin by scalp electrode.

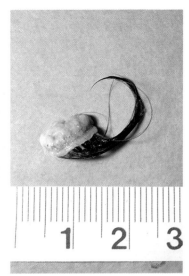

Fig. 229 Piece of avulsed skin.

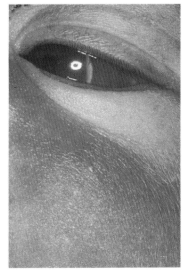

Fig. 230 Subconjunctival haemorrhage.

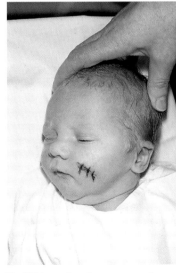

Fig. 231 Laceration at caesarean section.

Definition

The interval following labour taken to return to the normal non-pregnant state. Conventionally taken as 6 weeks, although most anatomical changes are complete within 2 weeks. In the UK it is a statutory requirement for mothers to be seen daily for 10–14 days by a midwife who routinely checks blood pressure, temperature, scars, lochia, breasts and involution of the uterus (Fig. 232), and also checks that the infant is well and advises on feeding difficulties.

General maternal complications

Puerperal sepsis: defined as a temperature of 38°C or more within 14 days of delivery. The usual causes include:
- breast infection
- urinary infection
- wound infection (if caesarean section)
- thrombophlebitis (legs or drip sites)
- thromboembolic disease
- pelvic infection (with or without retained tissue).

Perineum: perineal pain is extremely common following vaginal delivery and results from bruising (Fig. 233), oedema (Fig. 234) and infection. Analgesia, frequent bathing and removal of any tight sutures provide symptomatic relief. In more severe cases a course of perineal ultrasound may be beneficial.

Vaginal: vaginal haematomas (Fig. 235) are less common. Presentation is with increasingly severe pain in the rectum, usually within 6 h of delivery. The pain is often refractory to opiate analgesia, and the haematoma is palpable on vaginal or rectal examination. Management is by surgical evacuation of the clot, haemostasis and resuturing of the vagina and perineum. The amount of blood contained may be sufficient to make the patient anaemic. ➡

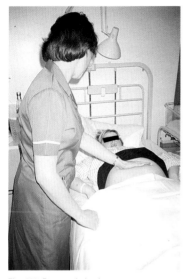

Fig. 232 Postnatal check.

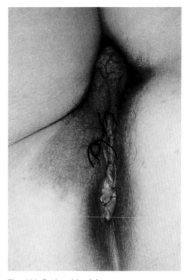

Fig. 233 Perineal bruising.

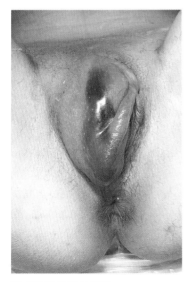

Fig. 234 Perineal oedema.

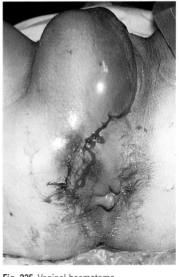

Fig. 235 Vaginal haematoma.

Haemorrhoids: a common complaint in pregnancy due to caval compression. They are prone to thrombosis and prolapse at delivery resulting in painful oedematous haemorrhoids (Fig. 236), a major source of puerperal discomfort. Management is by replacement of prolapsed haemorrhoids, analgesia (systemic and topical) and measures to prevent constipation.

Eyes: subconjunctival haemorrhages (Fig. 237) may result from maternal expulsive efforts during the second stage. They are symptomatic and resolve spontaneously.

Wound infection or haematoma (Fig. 238): follows in 10% of caesarean sections. They delay healing and when associated with a vertical incision, occasionally give rise to wound dehiscence (rare with transverse incision). Chest infection, thromboembolism, ileus, urinary tract infection and anaemia are also more common than following vaginal delivery.

Uterus: infection (endometritis) is usually at the placental site and presents with pyrexia, abdominal discomfort and vaginal bleeding. Treatment is with antibiotics and analgesia. Uterine rupture (Fig. 239) is fortunately rare, arising in about 1 in 2000 deliveries. Most ruptures occur during labour. In primigravidae rupture only occurs in association with previous uterine surgery, uterine manipulation or instrumental delivery. Multigravidae are more at risk, most ruptures occurring in a previous CS scar, especially vertical (classical) scars.

Deep venous thrombosis (DVT)/pulmonary embolus (PE):
PE is a leading cause of maternal mortality. More common in puerperium. DVT presents with pain in the leg or pelvis often with low grade pyrexia and leg oedema. PE often presents with pleuritic chest pain but there can be sudden collapse. If DVT or PE is suspected, i.v. heparinization should be commenced until diagnosis is refuted by venogram (DVT) or ventilation-perfusion scan (PE). ➡

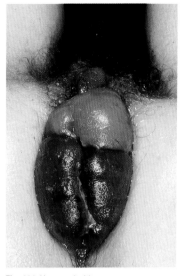

Fig. 236 Haemorrhoids.

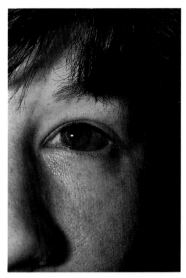

Fig. 237 Subconjunctival haemorrhages.

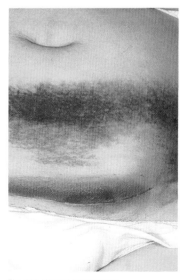

Fig. 238 Wound haematoma.

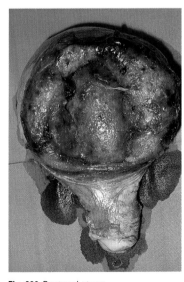

Fig. 239 Ruptured uterus.

Pituitary: postpartum necrosis of the anterior pituitary (Fig. 240) giving rise to Sheehan syndrome results from severe postpartum haemorrhage and shock. It is avoided by prompt management of haemorrhage, and now rarely occurs. The earliest presenting symptom is failure of lactation followed by amenorrhoea. Lifetime replacement of pituitary trophic hormones or those of their target organs is necessary.

Complications of breast-feeding

Engorgement of the breasts normally occurs on days 2 to 4. Mastitis (Fig. 241) is relatively common and starts with reddening and tenderness progressing to an oedematous induration with fever and malaise.

Aetiology

Staphylococci or streptococci, usually introduced by the baby during suckling, particularly on a cracked nipple, often with stasis of milk in a breast lobule or a blocked duct.

Management

Antibiotics (flucloxacillin), analgesics and regular emptying of the breast (infection is not a contraindication to continuing breast-feeding). Neglected mastitis will progress to abscess formation requiring surgical drainage. Drainage by aspiration using ultrasound guidance under local anaesthetic is preferable to incision of the breast.

Suppression

For mothers not wishing to breast-feed, firm support, avoidance of suckling and analgesia are usually sufficient. In circumstances where breast-feeding is contraindicated (e.g. following certain types of breast surgery, or in mothers who have experienced perinatal death), pharmacological suppression with bromocriptine tablets for 2 weeks may be indicated. Oestrogens are contraindicated because of the risk of thromboembolism.

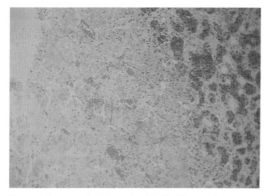

Fig. 240 Histology of pituitary gland in Sheehan syndrome.

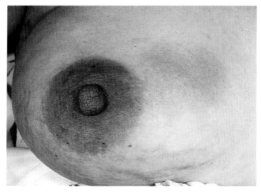

Fig. 241 Breast infection/mastitis.

Following pregnancy, sexual activity may be resumed once comfortable to do so, usually after a couple of weeks, by which time most anatomical changes of pregnancy have regressed. Return to fertility is variable and may be delayed for months by lactation. Non-lactating mothers may ovulate within 4 weeks of delivery and return of menstruation occurs on average at 58 days. It is extremely rare for fully breast feeding women to ovulate or menstruate prior to 10 weeks. Breast feeding alone, however, is not a reliable contraceptive method.

Success rate for any contraceptive method is documented as pregnancy rate per hundred women years (HWY) of usage. The first year of lactation/breast feeding with no other method has a failure rate of 10–20/HWY.

Hormonal methods

It is safe to use these in the puerperium bearing in mind the usual contraindications to use of oestrogen-containing preparations (including history of prior thromboembolism, cerebrovascular accident, hypertension or liver disease).

Types

Combined oestrogen/progestogen pills (Fig. 242): taken cyclically, they suppress gonadotrophins and should be started within 3 weeks of delivery if not breast-feeding, or when lactation ceases as they may suppress milk production. Blood pressure and weight are checked regularly and cervical cytology every 3–5 years (failure rate = <1/HWY).

Progestogen-only formulations (Fig. 243): no serious side effects, but they can cause menstrual irregularity. Oral progesterone preparations must be taken daily starting the second week after delivery. (Failure rate = <4/HWY.) Alternatively, depot-medroxyprogesterone acetate can be given by deep intramuscular injection lasting about 3 months. Once again irregular bleeding is a recognized side-effect (failure rate = <1/HWY).

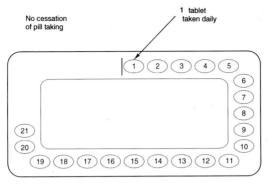

Fig. 242 Combined oestrogen/progestogen pill.

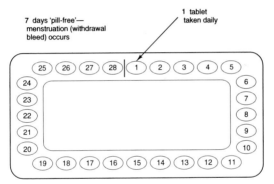

Fig. 243 Progestogen-only pill.

Intrauterine devices (IUD)

Insertion can be undertaken at any time in the puerperium. In general, however, expulsion rates are higher when insertion is earlier and thus, this is usually deferred until 6 weeks.

Insertion

A vaginal examination is first carried out to confirm the axis of the uterus (ante- or retroversion) and that it is of normal size. The cavity length is established with a uterine sound and the guard or the IUD introducer can be adjusted accordingly. The coil is introduced under aseptic technique. Sometimes it is necessary to grasp the cervix with a tenaculum.

Types

There are many varieties but they fall into three types: inert devices, those containing copper and a new levonorgestrel-containing device. Inert devices (Fig. 244) can be left in situ for many years but have more side-effects than do the smaller, copper-containing devices (Fig. 245). The latter also have slightly lower pregnancy rates but need to be changed every 2–3 years (failure rate = <4/HWY). The levonorgestrel coil has the main advantage of reducing menstrual flow, and a low incidence of pelvic infection. Its failure rate is comparable with female sterilization (see p. 143).

Complications

- Pelvic pain, menorrhagia and intermenstrual bleeding are common.
- Pelvic inflammatory disease is more common than with other methods of contraception.
- Uterine perforation. This probably occurs during insertion but usually only becomes apparent when the threads cannot be located subsequently. The location of the coil can be ascertained with ultrasound (Fig. 246) and surgical intervention may be necessary for removal.
- The rate of ectopic pregnancy is higher than with other methods, except possibly hormonal regimens containing only progestogen.
- Pregnancy. In the event of failure the spontaneous abortion rate is high.

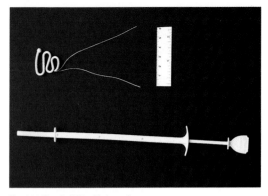

Fig. 244 Plastic IUD with introducer.

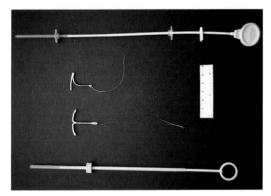

Fig. 245 Copper IUDs with introducer.

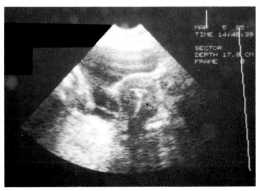

Fig. 246 IUD in situ on ultrasound (arrowed).

Barrier contraception

Unlike other methods, these offer some protection against sexually transmitted diseases; however, they have a slightly higher failure rate and additional use of spermicides is advisable as it improves their efficacy (failure rate = <15/HWY).

Types

Diaphragm (Fig. 247):   fits behind the cervix, covers it and is tucked up behind the symphysis pubis. The correct size needs to be assessed (often different after childbirth), and the patient taught to fit and check the diaphragm herself. It should be left in situ for several hours after intercourse.

Cervical cap: just covers the cervix and is similar, in principle, to the diaphragm.

Condom/sheath (Fig. 248):   a thin, rubber penile sheath with a reservoir to collect ejaculate or female equivalent for insertion into vagina.

Natural family planning

This requires self-recognition of ovulation by examination of cervical mucus and basal temperature. The changes of the puerperium and influence of lactation make such recognition difficult (failure rate = <30/HWY).

Sterilization

Only appropriate for those desiring permanent contraception. Tubal ligation or diathermy may be undertaken at the time of caesarean section or in the early puerperium (by minilaparotomy); however, the thickness and vascularity of the tubes at this time results in a higher failure rate. Delaying the procedure until after the puerperium enables laparoscopic sterilization at which a small portion of tube is occluded by application of a Silastic ring or clip (Fig. 249) (failure rate = <0.5/HWY).

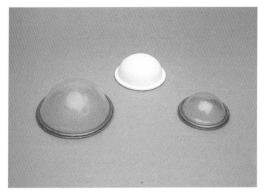

Fig. 247 Diaphragms.

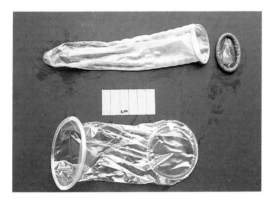

Fig. 248 Male and female condoms.

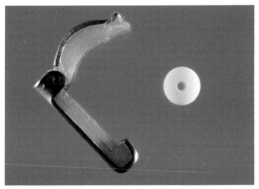

Fig. 249 Clip and ring for sterilization.

Index